Addressing Health Inequities in People With Serious Mental Illness

Addressing Health Inequities in People With Serious Mental Illness

A Call to Action

LEOPOLDO J. CABASSA

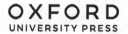

OXFORD
UNIVERSITY PRESS

OXFORD
UNIVERSITY PRESS

Oxford University Press is a department of the University of Oxford. It furthers
the University's objective of excellence in research, scholarship, and education
by publishing worldwide. Oxford is a registered trade mark of Oxford University
Press in the UK and certain other countries.

Published in the United States of America by Oxford University Press
198 Madison Avenue, New York, NY 10016, United States of America.

© Oxford University Press 2023

Library of Congress Cataloging-in-Publication Data
Names: Cabassa, Leopoldo J., author.
Title: Addressing health inequities in people with serious mental illness: a call to action/Leopoldo J. Cabassa.
Description: New York, NY, United States of America: Oxford University Press, [2023] |
Includes bibliographical references and index. |
Identifiers: LCCN 2022040755 (print) | LCCN 2022040756 (ebook) |
ISBN 9780190937300 (hb) | ISBN 9780190937324 (epub) | ISBN 9780197678947
Subjects: LCSH: Psychiatric social work—United States. |
Social Psychiatry—United States. | Mental health services—Social aspects. |
Social status—Health aspects. | Equality—Health aspects.
Classification: LCC HV690.U6 C33 2023 (print) | LCC HV690.U6 (ebook) |
DDC 362.2/04250973—dc23/eng/20221021
LC record available at https://lccn.loc.gov/2022040755
LC ebook record available at https://lccn.loc.gov/2022040756

DOI: 10.1093/oso/9780190937300.001.0001

1 3 5 7 9 8 6 4 2

Printed by Integrated Books International, United States of America

Contents

Preface

Two questions have shaped the work that my team and I have conducted over the past 10 years: Why do people with serious mental illness (SMI), like schizophrenia and bipolar disorder, die at an earlier age than those in the general population without these disorders? And what can be done to address this deadly health inequity? This book focuses on answering these two questions. It draws from existing research conducted by our team and others who are trying to disentangle the constellation of factors that shape the physical health of people with SMI and describes interventions, programs, and policies aimed at improving the health of this underserved and often marginalized population. The book goes beyond the data and the numbers and presents stories of people who live, struggle, and cope with SMI and physical health problems. It also tells the stories of clinicians, researchers, and policymakers who work to address these health inequities. In these pages, I strive to balance the presentation of scientific data, case studies, and personal narrative to raise awareness and foster compassion for this overlooked public health crisis and discuss ways to solve it.

My inspiration for this book comes from the experiences and the incredible people I met over the past 10 years as I ventured into this field of study as a Puerto Rican social work scholar and mental health services researcher. Through this professional and at times personal journey, I had the privilege to learn from, listen to, and bear witness to the struggles, hopes, and aspirations of people living with SMI and chronic medical conditions and the people who dedicate their lives to helping these populations. Given my professional dedication and calling for addressing racial and ethnic inequities in the delivery of health care and the fact that I come from a historically marginalized and colonized community in the United States, it was imperative that the work discussed in this book reflect the struggles, hopes, and aspirations of our diverse communities. Most of the stories represented in this book focus on historically marginalized and underserved racial and ethnic urban communities, mostly Blacks and Latino/as, that are often forgotten, excluded, and seriously underrepresented in the studies, trials, and policy discussions for improving the health of people with SMI.

Empathy is central to my work as a social work scholar. It entails step-ping into the world of others to understand their experiences without losing one's perspective and objectivity. The goal of my work is to use the scientific method with all its strengths and limitations to capture the lives of the people we are studying, to provide a voice to the voiceless, and to represent through numbers, stories, and analyses their needs, challenges, strengths, hopes, and dreams.

My approach to science has also been influenced by the work of Oliver Sacks, a physician, neuroscientist, and award-winning science writer who beautifully crafted case studies about people living with neurological disorders. A key element of his approach that has always resonated with my own work is the power of listening to the people we are studying and working with. As described by Dr. Sacks, clinicians and scientists often "underesti-mate the power of listening; it is by listening to our patients [participants and stakeholders] that we can discover their humanity. It is the only way to grasp what they are going through" (as quoted in Lehrer, 2007). Listening is "both engagement and research," understanding and action (Farmer, 2013, p. 20).

Through combining data and stories in this book, I intend to convey what people with SMI and chronic medical conditions are going through, to illus-trate the human side behind the often-cited statistics used to describe these health inequities. In the words of Dr. Luis Zayas, a senior colleague and mentor, "data cannot be allowed to eclipse the human" (Zayas, 2015, p. xv). Data and stories are both valuable as they reflect different phases of a phe-nomenon, the objective and the subjective, the detached and the engaged. By combining them we can grasp people's suffering and gain a better under-standing of what they are going through.

But we need to go beyond description. My work over the past 10 years has moved from knowing and understanding to application by formulating effective solutions and interventions grounded in people's needs and aspirations. This work focuses on applying what my team and I have learned from people's lives to develop, adapt, refine, test, and ultimately implement interventions that can make a positive impact in people's lives. The goal is to use knowledge to intervene by empowering the people we are trying to help with the knowledge, skills, resources, and confidence to improve their health and to develop interventions to help fix our fragmented and broken health care system.

The power of moving from understanding what people are going through to formulating a health intervention grounded on people's needs and

preferences was best encapsulated in a project we conducted several years ago in two supportive housing agencies in New York City (Cabassa et al., 2013). Supportive housing is an important service sector for reaching people with SMI in the community because these agencies provide affordable community-based housing alongside health, mental health, and social services. As part of a partnership between our team and these two agencies, we aimed to develop a project that enabled residents living in these agencies to discuss their physical health needs and generate ideas for potential health programs.

To capture what these residents were going through, we used a participatory research method called Photovoice in which participants are given cameras to document their lives around a specific topic and these photographs and the stories behind them are used to inform social action. This approach provides people the opportunity to use the power of the images they capture and the narratives that accompany these images to communicate their experiences and, via small group discussions, to formulate solutions to promote positive changes. As we described elsewhere, "The use of photographs, stories, and dialogues democratizes the knowledge-generation process, because it provides multiple mediums and opportunities for project participants to express themselves, represent their points of view, and communicate their ideas and reflections within a supportive environment" (Cabassa et al., 2013, p. 619).

This Photovoice project illustrates how using a participatory approach provides people with SMI an opportunity to have their voices heard and generate important insights about the type of health interventions they would prefer to address their health needs. This project produced concrete ideas about the format, content, and methods of health interventions for people in supportive housing. For example, residents described how they wanted health interventions that provided them with the knowledge and skills to improve their dietary habits by learning how to cook healthier meals for one person since most lived alone and did not want to waste food given their limited financial resources (Figure 0.1).

They talked about wanting a program that instead of telling them what to do showed them how to improve their health by providing them concrete strategies they could use in their everyday lives, for instance, how to shop for healthier foods on a tight monthly budget. They wanted the program to be delivered not by professionals but by people like them who had lived experiences recovering from SMI and working toward improving their

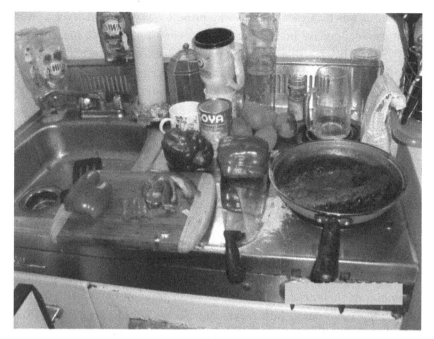

Figure 0.1 Participant's photo, titled "My everyday living."

Note: The participant's description of the photo was as follows: "It is really hard to cook for one. . . . For most of my life, I cooked for a family. I think that's why I'm having such a hard time now because I live alone now. And I haven't gotten that trick with just cooking for myself" (African American, male; Cabassa et al. 2013, p. 624).

physical health. This project planted the seed for a multiyear journey in which we used the lessons learned from these initial Photovoice discussions to develop a peer-led healthy lifestyle intervention for people with SMI in supportive housing agencies who are overweight or obese. We completed a large, randomized effectiveness trial testing the effectiveness and examining the implementation of this intervention in supportive housing agencies in New York City and Philadelphia (Cabassa et al., 2021; Cabassa et al., 2015).

As described more than a decade ago in an influential report titled *Morbidity and Mortality in People with Serious Mental Illness* written by the National Association of State Mental Health Program Directors, "There are multiple strategies to pursue in addressing morbidity and mortality. . . . But for any of these strategies to be successful, our principal partnership must be with the people we serve" (Parks et al., 2006, p. 32). To address health inequities among people living with SMI, particularly from racial and ethnic minoritized populations, we need to engage with communities, clients,

family members, and the stakeholders involved in serving this population to ensure that the programs, services, and policies we formulate to combat these inequities are fully responsive to the needs, preferences, and realities of our clients and their families. This book is inspired by what we have heard, what we have seen, and how we have used science and stories to help reduce these deadly health inequities.

Let's Clarify Some Terms

Several terms are used throughout the book that require some explanation and definition. The clarification of these terms will help orient readers about the topics and issues being discussed and how they relate to the physical health and health care of people with SMI.

First, a word on people with SMI—the people at the center of this book. SMI encompasses a cluster of mental disorders, such as schizophrenia spectrum disorders, bipolar disorder, major depression, and many others that interfere with major life activities, such as work, education, and social relationships, and cause serious functional limitations (Kessler et al., 2003; Substance Abuse and Mental Health Services Administration, 2017). Approximately more than 14.2 million adults 18 years of age or older in the United States reported an SMI in the past year, representing 5.6% of the U.S. adult population (Interdepartmental Serious Mental Illness Coordinating Committee, 2017; Substance Abuse and Mental Health Services Administration Center for Behavioral Health Statistics and Quality, 2014). These disorders are also costly since they represent five out of the 10 leading causes of disability worldwide (Vigo et al., 2016). People with SMI are overrepresented among the poor, those in disability programs, among those covered by Medicaid, and among those receiving services in the public mental health system (Alakeson et al., 2010; Castillo et al., 2017). They also consume a large proportion of the total Medicaid expenditures in the United States due to high rates of rehospitalization, use of emergency rooms, and high rates of comorbid physical health conditions like diabetes, cardiovascular disease, and cancer (Alakeson et al., 2010; Institute of Medicine, 2006). Despite these needs, recovery is possible for people with SMI with the appropriate resources, services, and supports. Of course, people with SMI are not a homogenous group. They are people with unique characteristics and strengths and diverse intersecting identities, histories, and backgrounds.

Second, what are health inequities? Health inequities are disproportionate and unfair differences in health outcomes such as the morbidity, mortality, prevalence, and incidence of disease that are caused by the interplay of behavioral, social, economic, political, and environmental disadvantages and "are often driven by the social conditions in which [people] live, learn, work, and play" (U.S. Department of Health and Human Services, 2017). For instance, compared to non-Hispanic Whites, Blacks have higher rates of heart disease, cancer, homicide, and diabetes (Kochanek et al., 2013). Inequities in health have "their roots in the structure of society and reflect the unequal life chances experienced by people of different social classes, racial/ethnic backgrounds, and other dimensions of social stratifications" (e.g., gender, age, geography, sexual orientation; Sampson et al., 2016, p. 517).

Third, we turn to health care inequities. Health care inequities are unfair differences between groups in the access to, use of, quality of, and outcomes of care despite no differences in their needs and preferences (Institute of Medicine, 2003). For example, historically marginalized racial and ethnic groups (e.g., Blacks, Hispanics, Native Americans) in the United States face numerous inequities in mental health care. Compared to non-Hispanic Whites, these populations are less likely to seek and receive care for common mental disorders (e.g., major depression, anxiety disorders), and when they do receive care they tend to drop out prematurely and receive care that is poor in quality (Institute of Medicine, 2003). Racial and ethnic inequities in mental health care persist even after controlling for educational levels, health insurance status, and mental health needs and result in greater persistence, severity, and burden of mental illness for racial and ethnic minoritized communities (Alegria et al., 2008; Institute of Medicine, 2003; Williams et al., 2007). Determinants of health care inequities include the operations and ecology of the health care system, legal and regulatory climate, and discrimination and biases (Institute of Medicine, 2003). In summary, inequities in health care arise because the providers, organizations, communities, and social institutions responsible for delivering health care fail to meet the needs of these historically marginalized populations due to a constellation of factors (e.g., cost, lack of culturally sensitive services, stigma, fragmentation of care; Cabassa, 2016).

Last, the events and stories related in this book are based on my memories and recollections of real-world events to the best of my abilities. To protect people's identities and to respect their privacy, I used fictitious names for most of the people represented in this book, with the exception of several

colleagues, clinicians, and researchers who provided permission to use their real names. Moreover, in the case examples I described throughout the book I altered personal details like place of birth, geographical location, age, gender, and medical histories to ensure their anonymity. The information from these case studies comes from our studies over the past 10 years and makes up a composite portrait of different people. Any resemblance to real people is purely coincidental and unintentional.

Acknowledgments

This book captures more than a decade of work. Many people contributed to the development of these ideas and have guided and supported me through this journey. Throughout my professional career, I have been fortunate to work alongside incredible mentors and senior colleagues such as Enola Proctor, Lawrence Palinkas, Lisa Dixon, John Landsverk, José Luchsinger, Shenyang Guo, Scott Stroup, Andrea Kriska, Melanie Wall, and Luis Zayas. Each have taught me invaluable lessons about social work, mental health services research, implementation science, and health equity research. I also want to thank Benjamin Druss for his mentorship in the early stages of my career and for opening the doors to learning about his work and the PCARE intervention. Ben's pioneering research and leadership for improving the physical health of people with serious mental illness (SMI) has always been an inspiration and a model for addressing these health inequities.

As special thanks goes out to Roberto Lewis-Fernández, who started me on this journey. Roberto, without your support, mentorship, collaboration, and encouragement, this work could not have been done. Many of the ideas presented in this book were planted, developed, and executed during our work at the New York State Psychiatric Institute's Center of Excellence for Cultural Competence (CECC) and during the many hours we spent traveling between New York City and Albany to support our center's work. Our time working together has been one of the highlights of my academic career. I still carry close to my heart the many lessons and skills I developed during my time at the CECC. *Mil gracias* for your unconditional support and mentorship. I have learned so much from you, particularly from your approach to science and the passion, integrity, and dedication you bring to your day-to-day work as a mental health services researcher, psychiatrist, and health equity scholar. I deeply value our collaboration and, most importantly, our friendship.

This work would not have been possible without the support and resources provided by my former Dean Dr. Mary McKay and my great colleagues, too many to name here, at the George Warren Brown School of Social Work and the Center for Mental Health Services Research at Washington University

in St. Louis. Thank you all for supporting this work and for providing me an academic home. Many of the projects described in this book were conceptualized and conducted while I was a faculty member at the Columbia University School of Social Work (CSSW). Thank you to all my great CSSW colleagues, especially Nabila El-Bassel, Jeannette Takamura, Julien Teitler, and Allen Zweben, who supported my work and encouraged me to push my ideas and science forward. A special shout-out to the CSSW crew, Carmela Alcántarra, Desmond Patton (now at University of Pennsylvania), Heidi Allen, and Courtney Cogburn—your work and dedication to rigorous social work science and social justice inspire me every day. Thank you for your support and friendship.

I would also like to thank the National Institute of Mental Health and the New York State Office of Mental Health for funding many of the studies presented in this book. A special thanks to Susan Azrin, David Chambers, and Lauren Hill from NIH for helping our team successfully navigate the NIH-funding process and for supporting our work. Thank you for all you do to improve the lives of people living with SMI and for supporting rigorous science to reduce health inequities in historically marginalized populations.

One of the great privileges of conducting this work is the opportunity to work alongside incredible students, early career investigators, clinicians, and peer specialists who bring incredible passion, dedication, and inspiration to this work. A special thanks to Nathaniel Lu, Morgan Dawkins, Sonika Aggarwal, Kechna Cadet, Talha Alvi, Kristen Gurdak, Katy Svehaug, Bailey Weir, Carolina Vélez-Grau, Arminda Gomez, David Camacho, Yamira Manrique, Michael Park, Lauren Bochicchio, Daniela Tuda, Mark Hawes, Nancy Pérez-Flores, Xiaoyan Wang, Kathleen O'Hara, Kellie Adams, Yonnie Harris, Lawrence Samuels, and Jeff Constantakis. Each of you contributed important insights to many of the studies presented in this book. This work would not have been possible without your hard work, dedication, and passion, often under difficult times and circumstances. To Mark Hawes, thank you for your thoughtful comments and edits to each of the chapters in this book.

I also owe a special thanks to the members of the community advisory board for the Bridges to Better Health and Wellness Intervention study: Quisqueya Meyreles, Lucia Capitelli, Richard Younge, Dianna Dragatsi, and Juana Alvarez. Your insights, expertise, and wisdom were critical for developing Bridges. I would also like to thank the staff and leadership at Bridges (Michael Blady), Pathways to Housing Philadelphia (Christine

Simiriglia and Lara Carson Weinstein), and Project Home (Monica Medina McCurdy) for opening your doors and for your invaluable work and support completing the Peer Group Lifestyle Balance (PGLB) project.

None of the work in this book would have been possible without the hard work, leadership, and dedication of Dr. Ana Stefancic, my most valuable collaborator and professional partner. Ana, I learned from you every day. You are a clear-headed, steady, and determined leader, an excellent scientist, and a dedicated and passionate advocate for improving the lives of people with SMI. The projects we conducted together have been an amazing journey with many ups and downs along the way, but all in all we have learned an enormous amount about the lives of people with SMI and how to work to improve the health of this population. None of this work would have been accomplished without your expertise, support, leadership, and friendship. Thank you from the bottom of my heart for the opportunity to work with you and to continue our collaboration.

I would also like to thank the scientists and clinicians I interviewed for this book, especially Stephen Bartels, Jackie Curtis, Kelley Aschbrenner, Gail Daumit, Mary Brunette, and John Newcomer. Thank you for your time and for sharing with me your stories. Your rigorous and innovative work is making a huge impact in improving the health and well-being of people with SMI. A special thanks to Michael McDonnell for reviewing the chapter on smoking and providing insightful edits.

Finally, thanks are due to my family: my mom, Eme; my big sister, Ana; and my dad, Leo (*que en paz descance*). Your unwavering support and unconditional love will always carry me forward. To my wife, Christine, your love, companionship, friendship, and support are what keep me going every day. Thank you for letting me bend your ear during our many walks, meals, car rides, and conversations about the ideas presented in this book. To my *nene*s, Leo Antonio and Vanessa, you are always my rock and support; I love you no matter what; your constant support inspires me every day.

Personal Note

My motivation for writing this book was not only academic or scientific in nature but also deeply personal. Living with mental illness and chronic diseases is a familial experience in my Puerto Rican family. Chronic diseases and psychiatric disorders have taken so much from both sides of my family. On my mother's side, we have experienced the ravages of cancer, diabetes, Parkinson disease, dementia, depression, heart disease, and suicide. My father's side is a similar story—these diseases have taken too many of my aunts and uncles. *Que en paz descancen*. I still carry close to my heart the last time I saw my beloved *Tio Tito* alive, my father's oldest brother. This man was full of life, love, and contradictions. He was a loving father of four, who could still get under my dad's skin, and was losing his battle against the cruelties of cancer. He knew his time was just around the corner, yet underneath his palpable fear, he seemed at peace with his family—my favorite aunt (I mean one of my favorite aunts) and my *primo* and three *primas*. That feeling of sadness engulfing their home for some reason has stayed imprinted on my heart, all these years later.

These personal experiences have shaped and informed whom, why, how, and what I study, shaping my professional and personal journey. As a Puerto Rican social work scholar, I rely on my family's experiences to ground my work and to never forget where I come from and whom my work represents. Social work has always appealed to me because it is an applied social science grounded in social justice values and goals. Our calling, training, mission, and professional ethics demand not only rigorous social and clinical sciences but also useful actions at all levels to inform the development and implementation of better treatments, programs, and policies to improve the quality of life and well-being of historically underserved, marginalized, and colonized communities. My experiences as a Puerto Rican scholar, husband, son, and father of two also ground the meaning and impetus of my work. I approached the work in this book not only with my academic training and scientific skills but also with all my *corazón* (heart).

1

"I'm Sick From Head to Toe"

> We know the reasons for this dreadful situation; we can no longer
> accept the consequences of twenty-five years lost because of our
> failure to act.
>
> —Carter (2010, p. 38)

Carla[1] had a schizoaffective disorder and multiple chronic medical
conditions when I first met her. At that time, she was participating in a series
of focus group discussions my team and I were conducting at a public outpatient mental health clinic in New York City to learn about the physical health
of Latino people living with serious mental illness (SMI; e.g., schizophrenia,
bipolar disorder) and their experiences seeking and receiving medical care.
Carla's story is typical of the people we met during our time at this clinic.

She was born in the Dominican Republic but had lived most of her life
in New York City. She spoke English and Spanish but preferred to talk in
Spanish with the patients and staff at the clinic. At the time of our project,
she was in her mid-40s living alone in a one-bedroom apartment in upper
Manhattan. She looked older for her age since she needed a cane to walk. She
had an adult daughter who came to visit her once or twice a week and helped
her get to her monthly appointments with her psychiatrist and social worker.
Her daughter often worried about Carla's health and tried to help in any way
she could by helping Carla with groceries and encouraging her to be more
physically active, but she had her own family and lived outside of the city.

During our group discussion, Carla described her health in the following
manner: "I'm sick from head to toe. I have many problems. I have diabetes,
high blood pressure; my mind is not right either. And I also have really bad
arthritis that I had for a long time." Carla visited a primary care clinic in her
neighborhood every 6 months but was not happy with the care she received
at this clinic. Like many participants in our group discussions, she described
the clinic as always full of patients with staff who seemed overburdened and

Addressing Health Inequities in People With Serious Mental Illness. Leopoldo J. Cabassa, Oxford University Press.
© Oxford University Press 2023. DOI: 10.1093/oso/9780190937300.003.0001

rushed. It took Carla 3 to 4 months just to get an appointment at this clinic, and once she arrived, she often waited hours to be seen by her doctor. Carla felt that she never had enough time with her doctor to discuss her medical conditions and to ask questions about her treatments.

Carla worried about all the medications she was taking, particularly the weight she had gained from her psychiatric medications. She knew this weight gain was bad for her health and making her diabetes and hypertension worse, but she did not have anyone to help her balance the treatments she was receiving for her health and mental health conditions. She mentioned that her primary care doctor and psychiatrist worried about her weight and deteriorating health and recommended that she lose weight, take her medication as prescribed, and take better care of herself, but provided little support or concrete strategies to accomplish these lofty goals.

During our group discussion, Carla talked about how she had tried many things over the years to address her health and mental health issues like dieting and trying to switch her psychiatric medications, but something always seemed to get in the way. Carla, along with other patients we met during our time at this clinic, mentioned how she had to stop dieting because it was too expensive for her to buy healthier foods: "Everything is so expensive," she said. "The things that are good for one are really expensive and one cannot buy everything." Carla's main source of income was her monthly disability check, which she needed to pay for more pressing issues like rent and utility bills. Carla felt resigned to being sick. She had lost confidence and trust in the health care system because of her negative experiences and poor health. Carla died of a stroke about a year after our group discussion.

Carla's description of her life exemplified many of the stories I heard time and time again over the past 10 years conducting studies on the physical health of people with SMI, particularly from the Black and Latino communities. In fact, I wrote Carla's words on a whiteboard at my office at the Columbia University School of Social Work and kept it there for years to remind me of the real human suffering and struggles behind the grim statistics we were studying. Carla died of preventable medical conditions that consumed her "from head to toe." Carla's untimely death, like the thousands of people with SMI who die each year in the United States from preventable and treatable medical conditions, is indicative of an ongoing national tragedy.

For more than half a century, the public health crisis impacting people with SMI has often been ignored and, until recently, rarely addressed. Compared

to people without mental disorders, people with SMI die at a younger age, between 8 and 30 years earlier depending on the studies you examine, largely due to preventable medical conditions like cardiovascular disease (CVD), cancer, and diabetes (Druss et al., 2011; Parks et al., 2006). This crisis is not new. The medical field has known about the premature mortality of people with SMI for decades.

One of the earliest reports in the literature published in 1937 in the *American Journal of Psychiatry* was conducted by Benjamin Malzberg from the New York State Department of Mental Hygiene (Malzberg, 1937). He found that psychiatric inpatients had a mortality rate approximately 6 times greater than the general population in New York State, largely attributed to "diseases of the heart" (p. 1327). In Europe, a similar mortality trend was reported in a study examining death rates in a Norwegian mental hospital from 1916 to 1941. According to Odegard (1951), men and women with schizophrenia had a mortality rate approximately 3 to 4 times higher than the general Norwegian population at that time.

Despite advances in health care and mental health treatments over the past half a century, people with SMI continue to die decades earlier than persons without these disorders. A series of factors have contributed to the poor physical health of people with SMI over the past 60 years. These include lack of national investments in the integration of health and behavioral health services, increasing rates of poverty among people with SMI, growing health and health care inequities in historically marginalized racial and ethnic communities, and the persistent stigmatization of people with SMI, to name a few. This deadly health inequity gained national attention in the United States in a landmark report published in 2006. In this report, Dr. Joe Parks and colleagues (2006) from the National Association of State Mental Health Program Directors examined mortality rates of people served in the public mental health system of eight states (Arizona, Missouri, Oklahoma, Rhode Island, Texas, Utah, Vermont, and Virginia). They found that people with SMI died, on average, 25 years earlier than the general population.

Premature mortality has also been found in people with SMI living in the community, not just those served in the public mental health system. A study led by Dr. Benjamin Druss and colleagues from Emory University, the University of Colorado, and the University of Pennsylvania examined mortality rates among people with mental disorders living in the community in a 17-year follow-up study using data from a nationally representative U.S. survey. For this study, they used data from the National Health

Interview Survey (NHIS), "the oldest and largest survey of the nation's health, administered annually since 1957" (Druss et al., 2011, p. 600). Druss and colleagues used data from the 1989 NHIS since it included a special supplement on mental health developed to estimate the prevalence of SMI in the United States (Barker et al., 1992). They then linked data from this supplement with the National Death Index mortality data for the subsequent 17 years to estimate and compare mortality rates between people with and without mental illness who participated in the 1989 NHIS study. They discovered that people with mental illness on average died 8 years earlier than people without mental illness. They also found that the average age at death dropped from 74 years for people with no mental disorders to 66 years for people with affective disorders to 64 years for people with substance abuse disorders to 63.4 years for people with psychotic disorders (Figure 1.1).

Similar trends in the premature mortality of people with mental disorders have been reported worldwide. A meta-analysis that pooled the results of 203 articles conducted in 29 countries across six continents found that the mortality of people with mental disorders, such as affective, anxiety, and psychotic disorders, was on average 2.2 times higher than that in the general population or people without mental disorders (Walker et al., 2015).

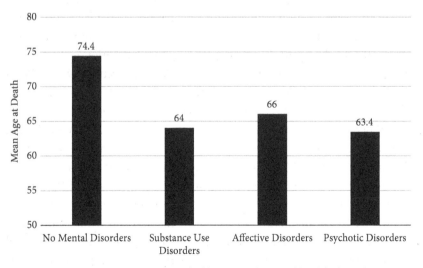

Figure 1.1 Mean age at death stratified by type of mental health disorder.
Note: Figure was orignially developed for this book presenting results reported in Druss et al. (2011).

More troublesome is evidence that the gap in mortality between people in the general community and persons with SMI, particularly those with schizophrenia, has been widening in the past decades. In a meta-analysis published in the *Archives of General Psychiatry* that included 37 studies conducted in 25 countries, Sukanta Saha and colleagues (2007) from the Queensland Centre for Mental Health Research and the University of Queensland found a steady linear increase in the standardized mortality ratio for people with schizophrenia throughout the 1970s, 1980s, and 1990s. The standardized mortality ratio (SMR)[2] is a measure that compares mortality rates between populations (e.g., people with schizophrenia versus people in the general population without schizophrenia) taking into consideration age and sex differences between these populations. For example, an SMR of 3 would mean that people with schizophrenia are 3 times more likely to die than people in the general population taking into consideration age and sex differences between these populations. Saha and colleagues (2007) observed that the SMRs for all causes of death among persons with schizophrenia increased from 1.84 in the 1970s to 2.98 in the 1980s to 3.20 in the 1990s. These findings suggest that people with SMI continue to experience excess mortality and have not benefited from improvements in health outcomes and life expectancy observed in the general population since the 1970s.

The population health implications of these findings are staggering. Mental disorders result in about 10 years of potential life lost and account for approximately 8 million deaths each year around the globe (Walker et al., 2015). People with mental illness die more often from unnatural causes, like suicide and injuries, than persons in the general population. But most deaths among people with SMI, approximately 67%, are due to natural causes such as CVD, cancer, diabetes, and other preventable medical conditions (Walker et al., 2015). These tend to be the leading causes of death and disability in the general population but are disproportionately common in people with SMI and tend to impact them at an earlier age. To illustrate these deadly health inequities, let's take a closer look at three major diseases linked to premature mortality in people with SMI: CVD, cancer, and diabetes.

Cardiovascular disease is a constellation of diseases that impacts the cardiovascular systems and the leading cause of death in the United States and in most Western developed countries (De Hert, Correll, et al., 2011). The World Health Organization (WHO) estimates that 17.9 million deaths worldwide, or 32% of all deaths, are attributable to CVD (WHO, 2021. In the United States and other developed countries, rates of CVD have been

declining due to improvements in prevention efforts and medical treatments and reductions in smoking rates. Despite these public health advancements, CVD continues to disproportionately impact people with SMI. Compared to people without mental disorders, the prevalence of CVD is approximately 2 to 3 times higher among people with schizophrenia, bipolar disorder, and major depression (De Hert, Correll, et al., 2011). The prevalence of CVD among people with SMI in the United States ranges from 4.8% to 55.3%, with an average of 22.7% (Janssen et al., 2015). CVD is the leading cause of death among people with SMI, killing them one to two decades earlier than people in the general population without mental disorders (De Hert, Correll, et al., 2011).

Cancer is a disease in which cells in the body grow out of control (Centers for Disease Control and Prevention [CDC], 2017a). It is the second leading cause of death worldwide (WHO, 2017a). Around the globe, approximately 8.8 million people died from cancer in 2015 (WHO, 2017a). In the United States, one out of every four deaths is attributed to cancer (CDC, 2017a). Cancer is also the second leading cause of death among people with SMI (Colton & Manderscheid, 2006). In a study examining premature mortality among people with schizophrenia covered by Medicaid in the United States, Olfson and colleagues (2015) found that people with schizophrenia were more likely to die of cancer (SMR = 1.8), particularly lung cancer (SMR = 2.4), than people in the general population. The prevalence of cancer among people with SMI in the United States ranges from 0.4% to 5.2%, with an average of 5.2% (Janssen et al., 2015). Multiple factors contribute to the higher mortality due to cancer in people with SMI, including advanced stage at presentation due to delays in diagnosis, barriers to screening and preventive efforts, complications in treatment due to the interaction of psychiatric and cancer medications, poor quality of care, and reduced access to specialized treatments (Weinstein et al., 2016).

Diabetes mellitus (DM) is a chronic disease that affects how the body extracts energy from the food we eat by either not making enough insulin or not being able to use the insulin our body already makes (CDC, 2017c). According to the CDC (2017c), approximately 30 million people in the United States have DM, which makes it the nation's seventh leading cause of death. DM is a major cause of adult blindness, kidney disease, heart attacks, stroke, and lower limb amputations (WHO, 2017b). Over the past 20 years, DM prevalence has risen rapidly in the United States and in middle- and low-income countries. The WHO (2017b) estimated that in 2014 422 million

people worldwide have DM. Compared to people without mental disorders, the prevalence of DM is approximately 2 to 3 times higher among people with SMI and is associated with reduced functioning and quality of life and premature mortality (De Hert, Correll, et al., 2011). The prevalence of DM in people with SMI in the United States ranges from 6.9% to 34%, with an average of 34% (Janssen et al., 2015). DM disproportionality impacts people with SMI, particularly in young adults (20 to 34 years old), elevating their risk for heart attacks, stroke, kidney failure, and amputations.

A constellation of factors impacts the excess morbidity and mortality associated with CVD, cancer, and diabetes in people with SMI. It includes the interplay of unhealthy behaviors, like higher rates of smoking and lack of physical activity; side effects of psychiatric medications, such as weight gain; detrimental social conditions that unfairly impact people with SMI, including high rates of poverty, stigmatization, unemployment, and homelessness; and the lack of access to high-quality medical care (De Hert, Correll, et al., 2011; Janssen et al., 2015). All can be prevented with appropriate treatments and programs, yet little has been done to reduce these deadly health inequities. Our health and mental health systems fail to act by not providing holistic and integrated care for health and mental health conditions, which contributes to this tragic public health crisis and has detrimental consequences in the lives of people with SMI and chronic medical illnesses, like Miguel.

Miguel was one of the first participants we recruited and interviewed in the same study in which I met Carla. At that time, he was in his mid-50s and receiving treatments for schizophrenia, diabetes, and high cholesterol. Miguel was a friendly and outgoing person eager to participate in our study and tell us his story. In fact, Miguel enrolled in our study because he truly wanted to do something to improve his health. He had seen other patients at the clinic suffer in silence with their health and mental health issues and did not want to end up being consumed by these illnesses and die before his time.

Miguel was born in Puerto Rico and moved to New York City in his teens. He was first diagnosed with schizophrenia in his early 20s and had been hospitalized multiple times since then. Each hospitalization was precipitated by his refusal to take his medications, which culminated in debilitating psychotic episodes marked by incessant auditory hallucinations and frightening visual hallucinations. Diabetes and high cholesterol came later in his life when he was in his late 30s, both of which were diagnosed during a psychiatric hospitalization.

Miguel was well liked by the social workers, psychiatrists, and staff at the outpatient mental health clinic where he had received care for years. He was always at the clinic helping in one way or another. The clinic served a daily lunch for patients, and Miguel always helped the kitchen staff with the dishes and other cleaning duties. He was not employed; his main source of income was his disability checks. He lived with his sister and brother-in-law in a small two-bedroom apartment in upper Manhattan. He did not like to stay home during the day, so the clinic became the center of his life, his home away from home. It was a place he felt safe, a place where he socialized with other people his age, with similar backgrounds and life experiences.

The best part of his daily routine between Mondays and Fridays was to play dominos after he completed his kitchen duties. There was always a steady group of regular patients at the clinic who stayed after lunch to play dominos in a small room the clinic had set up for the group. These were mostly men, but occasionally one or two women would also play or stay to watch and hang out. Like most people at this clinic, this group of patients came from the Caribbean, mostly Dominicans, Puerto Ricans, and a few Cubans. They usually played for a couple of hours, taking smoking breaks in between games and then going home around 3 p.m. depending on how the games went and people's schedules. It was a friendly but competitive group who enjoyed each other's company. Each game was filled with unrelenting bantering among the players and the people watching, all in good nature and fun.

The only times Miguel missed his routine at the clinic were the days he had an appointment with Dr. Rodriguez, his primary care doctor. Miguel had been going to this doctor for years. Dr. Rodriguez's clinic was always busy and had a long waiting list, but Miguel did not mind going there since he enjoyed seeing Dr. Rodriguez and trusted him. In fact, Miguel often joked that going to Dr. Rodriguez's was an all-day affair.

Miguel had been doing well managing his schizophrenia. He was taking his medications as prescribed and no longer felt the need to miss his medications. When we met, he had been out of the hospital for about a decade. He occasionally heard voices, but they came less frequently and did not seem to impact his everyday functioning. In many ways, after years of struggling with schizophrenia, he had finally reached a point where it did not consume him and did not threaten his stability. He knew he had to work at it, but he finally felt he had found a way to cope with this terrible illness.

His biggest concern now was his physical health. Miguel did not feel he was doing all he could to control his diabetes and high cholesterol. As he said

in one of our group discussions, "I am never at a 100%, it is not even an 80%, it is more like 70% or 65%. I take medicines, I inject my insulin, but it never feels like I'm getting better." His frustration stemmed from the fact that he knew what he needed to do in terms of taking his medications and insulin and going to his doctor. He also recognized that he needed to change his diet to eat more fruit and vegetables and less fast food, but he loved the fried foods from the bodegas in his neighborhood. He also knew he needed to engage in physical activity, but all he really liked to do was walk from his apartment to the clinic and back, several blocks each way. He had never done any sports or exercise in his life, so walking was all he knew how to do, but it was not enough.

In our group discussions, he expressed that he was fighting a losing battle and did not know what else he could do. He knew he needed more support and help but did not know where to go or even what that help would look like. His psychiatrist and social worker helped him with his schizophrenia. Dr. Rodriguez helped him with his diabetes and high cholesterol, but these clinicians rarely talked with each other and did not work together to support Miguel with his health issues. They rarely shared information about Miguel's conditions, medications, and treatments. It was left to Miguel to keep each provider informed about changes in medications and dosages and about results from laboratory tests, particularly for his glucose and cholesterol levels, and to inform each provider about each other's treatment plans. Miguel had to figure all this out on his own. He had to integrate the treatments he was getting for his schizophrenia with the treatments he was getting for his diabetes and high cholesterol. It would be a tough challenge for anyone, but even harder for someone with less than a high school education and living on disability payments.

This failure to integrate the treatments for mental disorders with the treatments for chronic medical conditions left Miguel in a serious and deadly bind. As we will see in later chapters, the gaps, inadequacies, neglect, and inefficiencies of the health care system greatly contribute to the excess morbidity and mortality seen in people with SMI. But, unlike Carla, Miguel's story did not end in tragedy. In fact, Miguel kept trying to figure this out with the tenacity and perseverance that he had used to recover from his schizophrenia. Several years later, he once again enrolled in one of our studies at a clinic where we trained social workers to be health care managers. I discuss this project in more detail later in this book, but Miguel benefited from having a social worker help him coordinate the care he was receiving for his

schizophrenia, diabetes, and high cholesterol and support him in being engaged in health behavior changes surrounding his daily dietary habits and physical activity. These behavior changes were not easy, but little by little, with support from his health care manager, Miguel was able to make the necessary adjustments to manage his health conditions.

The last time I talked with Miguel he was still enjoying his daily domino games at the clinic, but now he was no longer injecting insulin daily since his diabetes was better controlled, and his cholesterol was no longer elevated. Miguel had found a way with the right support, encouragement, and treatments to manage his battles against his health and mental health conditions.

At the heart of this book are people like Carla and Miguel, people living with SMI and chronic medical conditions that threaten them from "head to toe." In the following chapters, data and stories are combined to describe three key modifiable and urgent risk factors—unhealthy behaviors, side effects of psychiatric medications, and poor quality of medical care—that in combination contribute to the excess morbidity and mortality in people with SMI. We then move from risk factors to actions by describing several interventions that are used to reduce these risk factors and help improve the health of people like Carla and Miguel. Last, we end with a vision for the future by discussing research, practice, and policy recommendations for ending this public health crisis and for ending these deadly health inequities.

2

Cycles of Unhealthy Behaviors
in Unhealthy Environments

Our minds and bodies are deeply connected with each other. These interconnections influence what we do, how we feel, what we think, and how we behave, which in turn shapes our health and well-being. These linkages are critically important for the physical health of people with serious mental illness (SMI) since they shape health behaviors. What people with SMI eat; how much time they spend doing physical activity or being sedentary; whether they smoke, drink alcohol, or use drugs; and whether they take their medications as prescribed or go to the doctor are all health behaviors that directly influence their health status. Studying the health behaviors of people with SMI and the environmental factors that influence how these behaviors impact health are critical areas for understanding why people with SMI die earlier than the rest of the population. Beyond explanation, studying the health behaviors of people with SMI and their environments is also essential for the development of interventions and programs necessary to reduce these deadly health inequities.

I first began studying the connections between mental illness and chronic medical conditions during my time at the University of Southern California's (USC) School of Social Work, first as a postdoctoral fellow, and then as a newly hired assistant professor. During this time as an early career investigator, I conducted a qualitative study using a combination of focus group discussions and qualitative semistructured interviews to explore the illness experiences of Latino/a adults with diabetes and depression (Cabassa et al., 2008). This study was part of the Multi-faceted Depression and Diabetes Program for Hispanics, a randomized effectiveness trial funded by the National Institute of Mental Health (NIMH) and conducted in two public primary care clinics in Los Angeles, California (Ell et al., 2009). Kathleen Ell, a professor and colleague at USC, was the principal investigator of this trial.

As part of this qualitative study, we asked our Latino/a participants to talk about how their diabetes and depression related to each other and if these

Addressing Health Inequities in People With Serious Mental Illness. Leopoldo J. Cabassa, Oxford University Press.
© Oxford University Press 2023. DOI: 10.1093/oso/9780190937300.003.0002

conditions in any way influenced their everyday lives. The findings from this study, which we published in the journal *Social Science & Medicine*, provided a glimpse into the complex and reciprocal relationships between physical and mental illnesses, how deeply intertwined they are in people's lives, and how people cope with these conditions (Cabassa et al., 2008).

What we learned from this exploratory study was that participants tended to attribute their depression to the burden and loss of functioning linked to their diabetes. For these participants, the emergence of diabetes caused a series of losses in their everyday functioning that were meaningful to their lives, like their ability and capacity to work, take care of their families, and engage in daily activities. For many, these losses precipitated their depression. Participants also talked about how living with diabetes had an emotional impact in their lives. Many described how they struggled to adapt to the new demands imposed by their diabetes in terms of having to change their lifestyles (e.g., eating a healthier diet and increasing their physical activity) and follow diabetes treatments, like taking daily medications and/or insulin injections. Living in poverty further exacerbated these struggles and took an emotional toll for many participants that resulted in depression.

In turn, depression negatively influenced participants' engagement in the self-care behaviors needed to manage their diabetes. For example, participants talked about how changes in mood and motivation resulted in losing interest in caring for their diabetes, as described by a female participant: "When I fell into a depression I didn't care about the *azúcar* (sugar) because I even stopped eating, and I was very skinny" (Cabassa et al., 2008, p. 2418). Lastly, the very symptoms of diabetes (e.g., fluctuations in blood sugar levels) evoked, for some of our Latino participants, strong emotional reactions directly linked to their depression, such as having mood swings or feeling irritable, fatigued, or discouraged.

The experiences and findings from this early study propelled me to continue examining the multiple pathways by which health and mental illnesses impact one another, particularly how they influence people's health behaviors. Understanding people's illness experiences from their own perspectives is an important area of inquiry as it can help illuminate how people make sense of and attach meaning to these complex conditions, how they experience treatments, and how they cope with these chronic illnesses (Lopez & Guarnaccia, 2000). It provides a personal window into how people live and cope with these conditions. In the many focus groups and interviews my team and I have conducted with people with SMI since this

initial study at USC, we have continued to explore how people with SMI view the connections between their physical and mental health and how these connections shape their experiences living and coping with chronic medical conditions and mental illnesses.

Out of the many people who have participated in our studies, Rosa's answers to our questions have always stood out to me as she provided a vivid description of how her health and mental health were deeply interconnected and how these connections influenced her overall health. Her descriptions exemplified what we have learned from the many people with SMI whom we have studied over the years.

I met Rosa in the fall of 2011 in a public outpatient mental health clinic in New York City. At that time, Rosa was in treatment for major depression, hypertension, high cholesterol, and asthma. She was also a heavy smoker. Rosa was in her mid-50s when she enrolled in our study. She was born and raised in New York City and lived her entire life in upper Manhattan. Her dad was from Cuba and her mom was from Puerto Rico. She was bilingual and mixed English and Spanish seamlessly.

Her struggles with depression began in her mid-20s after a very difficult and painful divorce from an abusive husband. At that time, her ex-husband left her for another woman. After her divorce, she felt betrayed and alone and fell into a deep depression, not wanting to see or talk with anyone, wanting to be completely alone. She stopped talking to her friends and family members and stopped taking care of herself. Rosa talked about how she would spend days on end alone in her room watching TV and smoking. At times, she described how she did not even have the will to get out of bed. She also began to hear voices and see things. She felt confused and could not concentrate. She was terrified of what was happening to her.

Shortly after her divorce, she lost her apartment and moved in with her mother. Her mother was the one who finally convinced Rosa to go to the hospital to get help. Rosa talked about how her mother is the most important person in her life and her main source of companionship and support. Her mother helped her through several psychiatric hospitalizations by visiting her at the hospital and helping her connect to an outpatient mental health clinic where she felt welcomed and received the treatment she needed. When we met, Rosa had been attending the outpatient mental health clinic where we were conducting our study for the past several years. She liked that the clinic was nearby her mother's apartment, and that her psychiatrist and case manager were both female and very friendly.

During our interview, Rosa mentioned how her primary care doctor had recently expressed concern about her deteriorating health and worried that she was at high risk for a heart attack or stroke. Rosa was very concerned about this and knew that her dietary habits, lack of exercise, and smoking were contributing to her poor health. She wanted to change these unhealthy behaviors but did not know how. When I asked her whether she saw any connections between her health and mental health, Rosa answered:

> If you have a problem with depression, you eat . . . or smoke . . . and it affects your heart. So, your heart and your obesity says to your mind: listen, I'm eating a lot or it affects your cholesterol or it affects your sugar . . . you feel fat and ugly . . . so that affects your mind . . . from there comes the depression to eat more. The circle comes again to eat more and smoke more and have more dependency on other things.

Rosa also talked about how this cycle can start from health issues. Like other people we interviewed, Rosa was bothered by pain, particularly in her lower back and knees. She mentioned how pain frequently interfered with her everyday functioning and her motivation to engage in pleasurable activities, like going out with friends or taking a walk at a nearby park, which in turn led to isolation and frustration, fueling her mental health symptoms, particularly her depression. This cycle exemplified how physical health issues contributed to her depression, and during really bad times she described how it "depleted her will to do things."

Rosa's experiences illustrate how negative connections between her physical and mental illnesses can result in poor health. What we learned from Rosa is that her illnesses are not separate entities. Her conditions impacted each other in complex and often negative ways, resulting in reinforcing cycles of unhealthy behaviors that were difficult to break. These cycles provide fertile ground for chronic illnesses to take hold and flourish. Rosa's experiences also captured how these cycles can begin from multiple places. They can begin from the physical health side or from the cascade of symptoms associated with SMI, particularly those linked to motivation, mood, cognition, and energy that deplete people's volition. Regardless of where these cycles begin, they give rise to unhealthy behavioral patterns that become negative health habits if left untreated or ignored.

The significance of these unhealthy cycles of behaviors in people with SMI is that they are directly linked to the health conditions (e.g., diabetes,

cardiovascular disease, cancer) that are disproportionally prevalent in this population. In fact, these health behaviors, often characterized as lifestyle factors, are significant determinants of the physical health of people with SMI, accounting for most of the excess mortality in people with mental disorders (Druss et al., 2011). According to the World Health Organization, an estimated 80% of premature mortality due to cardiovascular disease (CVD), the leading cause of death in people with SMI, is attributed to the perfect yet deadly storm of sedentary lifestyle, low levels of physical activity, poor dietary habits, and high rates of smoking (World Health Organization, 2002). All, as we will see, are common in people with SMI.

Sedentary behaviors, like sleeping, sitting, or watching TV, are activities with low energy expenditures (Vancampfort et al., 2012). Compared to people without mental illness, people with SMI tend to spend significantly more time engaged in sedentary behaviors. Dr. Brendon Stubbs from Kings College in London published in 2016 one of the first systematic literature reviews and meta-analysis examining sedentary behaviors in people with SMI (Stubbs, Williams et al., 2016). Based on their examination of 13 articles that included 2,033 participants, they estimated that on average people with psychosis spend 11 hours per day being sedentary, which is approximately 3 extra hours of sedentary behavior compared to people in the general population without psychosis (Stubbs, Williams et al., 2016). They concluded that the time people with psychosis spend being sedentary is one of the highest compared to other populations (e.g., people in the general population) reported in the literature. These findings illustrate an alarming, unhealthy pattern among people with SMI because sedentary behaviors are linked to poor health outcomes and premature mortality. Among people with SMI, these behaviors are significant predictors of body mass index (BMI) and the metabolic syndrome, a cluster of conditions (e.g., high blood pressure, excess body fat around the waist, elevated levels of cholesterol) that increases a person's risk of CVD, stroke, and diabetes (Vancampfort et al., 2012).

On top of being more sedentary, people with SMI tend to be less physically active than people who do not have mental illness. A recent meta-analysis of 35 studies examining different levels of physical activity in people with schizophrenia, also conducted by Brandon Stubbs and colleagues, estimated that people with schizophrenia engage in significantly less moderate and vigorous physical activity when compared to people without mental illness (Stubbs, Firth et al., 2016). For example, they found that people with schizophrenia on average spend 14.2 minutes less in moderate physical activity per day when

compared to healthy controls. The U.S. Surgeon General recommends that adults engage in 150 minutes per week of at least moderate-intensity activity, meaning physical activity that makes people breathe harder than normal, like when going on a brisk walk or bicycling. About half of people in the general population (53%) meet this physical activity recommendation (Centers for Disease Control and Prevention, 2017b). Yet, the proportion of people with SMI that meet this guideline for physical activity is much smaller, about 25% in some studies (Faulkner et al., 2006). These high levels of sedentary behaviors and low levels of physical activity are troublesome trends in people with SMI since each are independent risk factors for diabetes, CVD, and cancer (Biswas et al., 2015). All are conditions that directly contribute to premature death in people with SMI.

Add to these a poor diet, smoking, and substance use disorders, and you have the perfect kindling fueling the development of chronic medical conditions and poor health outcomes in people with SMI. People with SMI tend to have poor dietary habits compared to people without these disorders. For example, in one of the few systematic literature reviews examining the dietary patterns of people with SMI, Dr. Salvatore Dipasquale and colleagues (2013) from the Institute of Psychiatry at King's College reported that people with schizophrenia were more likely to consume a diet low in fiber and fruits and rich in saturated fats compared to people without schizophrenia. This type of diet increases the risk of developing metabolic abnormalities, including obesity, high cholesterol, and increased fasting glucose. All elevate the risk for CVD and diabetes.

People with SMI are also more likely to smoke and to be heavy smokers, meaning that they smoke at least 25 cigarettes a day, compared to people in the general population (Campion et al., 2008; Ziedonis et al., 2008). As many as 80% of people with schizophrenia use tobacco products in comparison to only 20% to 23% in the general population (Parks et al., 2006; Ziedonis et al., 2008). More troublesome is that people with a mental illness in the past month consumed nearly half (~44%) of all cigarettes sold in the United States (Lasser et al., 2000). Reducing smoking among people with SMI is the "intervention that is likely to have the greatest impact on decreasing mortality" since smoking is directly linked to the leading causes of death (CVD and cancer) in people with SMI (Parks et al., 2006, p. 17).

Lastly, the abuse of substances, like alcohol, cannabis, opioids, cocaine, and others, is common in people with SMI. It is estimated that a quarter of adults 18 years of age or older with SMI (25.4%), about 2.6 million people,

report a substance use disorder in the past year (Interdepartmental Serious Mental Illness Coordinating Committee, 2017). It is estimated that among people with SMI who also have a comorbid substance use disorder, one in six has abused opioids (16%), and one in 10 (10%) has abused alcohol in the past year (Interdepartmental Serious Mental Illness Coordinating Committee, 2017; Koskinen et al., 2009). If left untreated, substance abuse in people with SMI has a profound impact on every aspect of the person's health, course of illness, functioning, quality of life, and clinical care. For example, early mortality is higher in people with SMI who have a substance use disorder than those without, particularly among people with SMI who abuse alcohol and drugs like opioids, cocaine, stimulants, hallucinogens, and volatile solvents (Hjorthoj et al., 2015). Substance use disorders in people with SMI are also linked to higher levels of incarceration, more frequent hospitalizations and relapse, more severe symptoms, poorer course of illness, higher rates of homelessness and suicide, and increased health care costs (Bellack et al., 2006; Interdepartmental Serious Mental Illness Coordinating Committee, 2017). Preventing and treating substance use disorders in people with SMI are critical to improving the health, well-being, and overall quality of life of this population.

As we have seen with Rosa's experience and in the discussion of unhealthy lifestyles of people with SMI, these behaviors are linked to poor health and early mortality, but they do not happen in a vacuum. What people with SMI do, the choices they make regarding their diets, their physical activity, and whether they smoke or use substances are influenced by their environment, by the world that surrounds them. A person's health is intimately connected to their environment. To better understand and, ultimately, improve the health behaviors of people with SMI, we also need to understand where they live, work, and play; how they cope with stress in their everyday lives; their social interactions and cultural norms; and how they navigate these contexts.

The importance of context in the health of people with SMI became apparent in one of the first studies I got involved in after I left USC and began a new position at the New York State Psychiatric Institute (NYSPI) and at the Department of Psychiatry at Columbia University. At that time, the team that I was joining as the assistant director of the New York State Center of Excellence for Cultural Competence at the NYSPI was conducting a large qualitative study in six behavioral health organizations (e.g., outpatient mental health clinics, supportive housing programs) in upper Manhattan, particularly in the neighborhoods of Harlem, Washington Heights, and

Inwood, serving racial and ethnic minoritized people with SMI, predominantly Black and Latino/a adults (Cabassa, Siantz et al., 2014). We wanted to learn from different stakeholders (e.g., administrators, providers, clients, and their family members) how these organizations were addressing the physical health needs of these diverse clients, what factors influence the health of this population, and what could be done to improve the health of these historically underserved and marginalized communities. We used a combination of qualitative methods to collect these data, including individual semistructured qualitative interviews, focus group discussions, and participant observations. We published the results of this study in two papers, one in *Qualitative Health Research* and the other in the *Journal of Health Care for the Poor and Underserved* (Cabassa, Siantz, Nicasio et al., 2014; Ezell et al., 2013).

Three findings from these publications illustrate how context can shape the health behaviors of people with SMI, particularly around dietary choices and physical activity. First, food environments, "the structure, type, density, and proximity of food outlets," is an important contextual determinant of health (Cannuscio et al., 2010, p. 382). Many people with SMI, including the people we interviewed in our study, live in neighborhoods with unhealthy food environments where healthy foods, like fresh fruits and vegetables, are unavailable and unaffordable. Their neighborhoods are also characterized by a high density and accessibility of fast-food establishments and bodegas (corner stores) that serve limited nutritional foods. The socioeconomic status of people with SMI further compounds the problems of living in an unhealthy food environment. Many people with SMI live in poverty and rely on disability payments as their main source of income, thus restricting their dietary options, as described by this clinic administrator we interviewed: "What's in the neighborhood? What do you have access to? What can you afford to pay for? For a lot of our patients [referring to people with SMI served at her organization], it's not practical for them to prepare their own foods because they may not have access to a kitchen, or they may not be cognitively with it and want to cook their own food, so it's easier to go to McDonald's and just buy a Big Mac, than to go buy a chicken and cook it and season it. The nutritional needs of our patients are high, [but] it's not just what they put in their mouths, it's what they have access to" (Ezell et al., 2013, p. 1560).

Furthermore, what a person can and cannot afford shapes the choices they make when shopping for food, even when they know they are making

unhealthy choices. As we learned from our participants, limited financial resources create serious constraints in their diets, as described by a Black participant with SMI:

> If you don't have enough money . . . you buy foods that are really not good for you. . . . You want to buy a bag of oranges, but a bag of oranges is not going to last that long. There are bags of potato chips . . . [that] are going to last longer. They are cheaper. You go for what's cheaper, what's going to last longer . . . and you can't afford that extra expense of better foods. (Cabassa, Siantz, Nicasio et al., 2014, pp. 1131–1132)

Second, cultural and social norms influence dietary choices. Our views, attitudes, beliefs, and habits about food and dietary practices are shaped by our culture, by what we learn from family members, friends, professionals (e.g., doctors), coworkers, and the marketing messages from the food and beverage industries. A surprising finding in our study was that many of the Latino/a and Black clients with SMI who participated in our study had internalized the view that racial and ethnic minorities live unhealthy lives because of their diets and traditional foods, as captured by this Latina participant with SMI: "We lead very unhealthy lives . . . I mean, with the Spanish, you know with all that rice and beans and all that seasoning" (Cabassa, Siantz, Nicasio et al., 2014, p. 1132). A leader in the Black community we interviewed also expressed this same sentiment: "Like, how do we educate ourselves to cook collard greens differently? And not smother pork chops . . . to know that we don't have to have fried chicken and cornbread and green beans, we don't have to have all of this" (Cabassa, Siantz, Nicasio et al., 2014, p. 1132).

As discussed in our publications of this study, this self-blame and these negative views about traditional diets suggest that some racial and ethnic minoritized people with SMI may

> internalize a racist view that devalues traditional foods and practices as generally unhealthy, when in fact traditional cuisines are full of time-honored healthy food choices. Explicit consumerism and targeted food marketing to minority communities could contribute to the internalization of self-blame by supporting the view that traditional foods are less valuable compared to modern, dominant-culture dietary options, such as fast-foods. (Cabassa, Siantz, Nicasio et al., 2014, p. 1134)

Our findings suggest that changing unhealthy cycles of behaviors requires attention to cultural and social norms. What we eat is deeply embedded in our cultural identity and the social norms that surround our dietary practices. Interventions and programs that aim to help people with SMI improve their diets must take culture into consideration. For example, sessions and specific modules in these programs can include recipes and show participants how to prepare their traditional foods in a healthy manner without compromising taste (Cabassa, Siantz, Nicasio et al., 2014).

Third, engagement in physical activity requires access to safe and accessible environments, like parks, bike lanes, pedestrian walkways, and affordable gym memberships. Many of the people we talked to in this study reported that lack of access to safe environments deterred many people with SMI from engaging in regular physical activity, as described by this Latina with SMI: "I do not feel comfortable walking alone in the streets. . . . I get very nervous" (Cabassa, Siantz, Nicasio et al., 2014, p. 1133).

In all, the health of people with SMI is shaped by unhealthy behaviors in unhealthy environments that require not only behavioral change strategies to break these unhealthy habits but also structural changes to their environments. We need multifaceted approaches that help people with SMI while at the same time changing their environment. Interventions need to address people's views, attitudes, and knowledge about their health behaviors; empower them with the behavioral skills necessary to create positive health habits; and create local social worlds that are supportive of healthy lifestyles. These are lofty goals, and more work is needed to create better interventions, programs, and policies that are responsive to the needs, preferences, realities, and environments of people with SMI from all cultural backgrounds (Cabassa Siantz, Nicasio et al., 2014). This work will require resources, changes in practices, motivation, and commitment from multiple stakeholders, but as we will see in future chapters, it can be accomplished.

3

"It Cures You in One Way and It Damages You in Another"

In almost every interview and focus group discussion we have conducted examining the health of people with serious mental illness (SMI), the topic of psychiatric medications, particularly second-generation antipsychotics, always finds its way into the conversation. As captured by the title of this chapter, our participants, time and time again, voiced serious concerns about taking these medications, especially around issues of weight gain and fears that these medications may increase their risk for developing chronic medical illnesses.

Second-generation antipsychotics, such as olanzapine, risperidone, and quetiapine, are important for treating people with SMI. These medications help reduce symptoms, restore and improve functioning, prevent relapse, and provide many people with SMI a pathway to recovery (Correll et al., 2018). A key advancement of second-generation antipsychotics is that they do not produce the neurologic extrapyramidal side effects (e.g., body rigidity, involuntary tremors, akathisia, tardive dyskinesia) associated with first-generation antipsychotics like haloperidol (American Diabetes Association [ADA] et al., 2004). These side effects make first-generation antipsychotics intolerable for many people, resulting in diminished functioning and treatment nonadherence (ADA et al., 2004).

Yet, second-generation antipsychotics are not without side effects. These medications produce health side effects, such as weight gain, and increase cardiometabolic abnormalities, such as elevated lipid and fasting glucose levels, which, when ignored, unmanaged, or left untreated, can cause serious health consequences. These adverse effects increase the risk for obesity, type 2 diabetes, dyslipidemia, metabolic syndrome, and ultimately cardiovascular disease (CVD; De Hert, Detraux et al., 2011). These cardiometabolic side effects create a difficult quandary for people taking these medications because they are forced to choose their mental well-being at the expense of their physical health. A person with SMI taking these medications should

Addressing Health Inequities in People With Serious Mental Illness. Leopoldo J. Cabassa, Oxford University Press.
© Oxford University Press 2023. DOI: 10.1093/oso/9780190937300.003.0003

not have to live a lifetime of physical illness to achieve good mental health ("No Mental Health Without Physical Health," 2011). Enrique's experiences exemplify this dilemma.

Enrique was in his mid-20s when we first met him several years ago as a participant in one of our studies. He described himself as Afro-Caribbean because his mother was African American and his father was Dominican. Enrique was born and raised in New York City. He felt most comfortable speaking English, although he understood Spanish very well. He was diagnosed with schizophrenia in his early 20s after a series of psychotic episodes in which he heard voices telling him to harm himself. Each episode resulted in a psychiatric hospitalization where he was given a second-generation antipsychotic to help stabilize his condition. The medication helped reduce the voices, and he was able to return home and resume his life. When we met, he was receiving outpatient mental health services at a local public mental health clinic.

Enrique had been taking Zyprexa for a couple of years and felt that it helped control the voices in his head, but it came at a cost that deeply concerned him. During our focus group discussion, he related that he had "gained [a] tremendous amount of weight" and felt like the medication zapped his energy and motivation. On Zyprexa, he told the group, "I had no energy. I had no interest in doing any type of activity, apart from staying home." He knew this medication helped and was necessary to keep him out of the hospital, but it had started to affect his physical health. When we met, he had just gotten news from his primary care doctor that he had high cholesterol and that his body mass index (BMI) was now in the obese range. This concerned him, and he worried about what this medication was doing to his body. He did not want to end up with a chronic medical condition so early in his life. He felt conflicted and did not know what to do. Zyprexa was helping him with his mental health, but it came at the expense of his physical health. He summarized this dilemma in the following way: "It cures you in one way and it damages you in another." His health concerns were real. If they were not properly addressed, Enrique's weight gain and high cholesterol could result in a trajectory of poor health outcomes and potentially premature mortality.

As illustrated by Enrique's case, weight gain is a well-established side effect of second-generation antipsychotic medications. Approximately 15% to 72% of people with schizophrenia receiving treatments with antipsychotic medications experience substantial weight gain (De Hert, Detraux, et al., 2011). Weight gain is an undesirable consequence of taking these

medications and can result in stress, negative self-esteem, problems with interpersonal relationships, poor health, and treatment discontinuation (Gentile, 2006). For instance, in the Clinical Antipsychotic Trials of Intervention Effectiveness (CATIE), one of the largest double-blind clinical trials testing the effectiveness of antipsychotic medications, which enrolled 1,493 adults with chronic schizophrenia from 57 clinical sites in the United States, weight gain was one of the most common reasons for participants to discontinue treatment, particularly among those randomized to receive olanzapine (Lieberman et al., 2005).

The mechanisms explaining antipsychotic-induced weight gain are complex and not completely understood (ADA et al., 2004). In its most basic form, weight gain results when a person's energy intake supersedes their energy expenditures, meaning a person consumes more calories than they burn. There is some evidence that the weight gain related to the use of antipsychotic medications may be due to mechanisms related to appetite stimulation because these medications interact with several of the brain's receptors involved in appetite regulation (e.g., histamine H_1, 5-HT_{2c} receptor; De Hert et al., 2009).

Not all antipsychotic medications produce the same amount of weight gain. In fact, there are important differences between these medications that can inform clinical decisions. For example, results of clinical trials examining weight gains after 10 weeks of treatment indicate that clozapine and olanzapine produce the largest amount of weight gain (4.45 kg and 4.15 kg, respectively) followed by quetiapine and risperidone (2.1 kg), with aripiprazole and ziprasidone reporting the least amount of weight gain (< 1 kg; De Hert et al., 2009). Similar differences in the weight gain propensity of second-generation antipsychotic medications have been found when examining longer periods of treatment (e.g., over a year; Gentile, 2006; Newcomer & Haupt, 2006) and among children and adolescents first exposed to these medications (Correll et al., 2009).

Weight gain seems to occur more rapidly in the first year of treatment and then it tends slow down (Allison et al., 2009). However, long-term progressive increases in weight have been reported (Gentile, 2006). Based on the existing evidence from multiple clinical and observational studies, all antipsychotic medications, either first or second generation, are related to some level of weight gain because the percentage of people who experience clinically significant weight gain—defined as gaining 7% or more of their pretreatment weight—tends to be consistently greater among people taking

these medications compared to people taking placebos (De Hert, Detraux, et al., 2011).

On top of weight gain, second-generation antipsychotic medications produce serious cardiometabolic side effects, particularly those associated with metabolic syndrome (Correll et al., 2015; De Hert, Detraux, et al., 2011). This syndrome consists of a constellation of abnormalities including central obesity, hypertension, dyslipidemia, glucose intolerance, and insulin resistance, which significantly increase the risk for CVD, stroke, diabetes mellitus, and premature mortality (De Hert, Detraux, et al., 2011; Mitchell et al., 2013). Metabolic syndrome is prevalent among people with SMI. In a meta-analysis of 77 publications that included a total of 25,692 people with schizophrenia drawn from 27 countries or regions, Alex Mitchell and colleagues (2013), from the University of Leicester in the United Kingdom, found that one in three people with schizophrenia suffered from metabolic syndrome, one in two was overweight, one in five was prediabetic, and approximately two in five had lipid abnormalities. They also reported that the highest rates of metabolic syndrome were seen in people prescribed olanzapine (51.9%), and the lowest rates were seen among people who were not medicated (20.2%; Mitchell et al., 2013). Moreover, the risk for cardiometabolic abnormalities seems to be higher among people with schizophrenia in later stages of their illness compared to people with first-episode psychosis and among those with schizophrenia who are drug naïve, meaning they have previously not received antipsychotic medications for their illness (Mitchell et al., 2013; Vancampfort et al., 2013).

The physical health concerns surrounding the use of second-generation antipsychotics have prompted patients, family members, advocates, and mental health professionals alike to question the safety of these medications and why more has not been done to identify and counteract these health side effects. These concerns have resulted in the filing of multiple lawsuits against pharmaceutical companies that developed and marketed these drugs. A well-known series of cases are the ones against Eli Lilly, the developers of Zyprexa (olanzapine), for its misrepresentation of this commonly used antipsychotic medication. Internal Eli Lilly documents that came to light during multiple lawsuits uncovered how this company downplayed the cardiometabolic side effects of Zyprexa when marketing this medication to doctors by not properly disclosing data on weight gain and high blood sugar levels from their internal clinical trials (Berenson, 2007). For instance, court documents showed that Eli Lilly's marketing materials used to inform doctors about Zyprexa's

benefits and side effects failed to disclose that patients participating in the company's clinical trials and randomized to take Zyprexa were 3.5 times more likely to experience high blood sugar levels than those randomized to placebo (Berenson, 2006a). Moreover, internal Eli Lilly memos showed that data from its clinical trials used in their marketing materials had been intentionally misrepresented to downplay Zyprexa's side effects (Berenson, 2006a). Instead of disclosing that the incidence of treatment-emergent hyperglycemia in the Zyprexa group was 3.6% compared to 1.05% in the placebo, the information presented to doctors painted a different picture (Berenson, 2006a). It reduced the risk in the Zyprexa group to 3.1% and increased the risk in the placebo group to 2.5%, thus suggesting that the risk of treatment-emergent hyperglycemia was similar between the two groups (Berenson, 2006a).

These documents also showed that the company marketed Zyprexa for other conditions not approved by the Federal Drug Administration (FDA), such as for symptoms of dementia, and that it targeted primary care doctors to dispense this powerful antipsychotic medication for off-label conditions (Berenson, 2006b). Zyprexa is not approved to treat dementia, nor any psychotic symptoms related to dementia. In fact, this medication carries a "prominent warning from the F.D.A. that it increases the risk of death in older patients with dementia-related psychosis" (Berenson, 2006b). In January 2007, Eli Lilly paid $500 million to settle 18,000 lawsuits from patients claiming that Zyprexa caused their diabetes and other chronic diseases (Berenson, 2007). These payments came on top of earlier settlements over Zyprexa of $1.2 billion to 28,600 plaintiffs claiming they were injured by this medication (Berenson, 2007). Numerous lawsuits are still pending in state and federal courts.

The cases against Eli Lilly illustrate a troublesome reality within the pharmaceutical industry in which profits come before the overall well-being of vulnerable patients. Second-generation antipsychotics are critical for helping people with SMI, but they do have serious health side effects that cannot be ignored, misrepresented, or downplayed, as shown in Eli Lilly's marketing practices. No medication is perfect, but not alerting doctors who prescribe these medications and the people who take them about their potential side effects is criminal and unethical. Doctors, patients, family members, and the public at large have the right to know both the benefits and risks of taking these medications so that an appropriate treatment choice can be made and efforts to screen and mitigate side effects can be addressed. In people

with SMI, the lack of attention to the health side effects of antipsychotic medications by the makers of these compounds has contributed to their poor health outcomes and deadly health trajectories.

Given that second-generation antipsychotic medications continue to be a common and widely prescribed treatment for people with SMI and are associated with multiple cardiometabolic side effects, it is imperative to understand the long-term health consequences of these medications. These consequences are not easy to study. Doing so requires large, diverse, and representative samples of people with SMI and longitudinal designs that follow people over a long period. It also requires rigorous methodological and analytical techniques to control for common biases, like differential adherence rates, dose effects, psychiatric illness severity, functional impairments, BMI, unhealthy lifestyle behaviors (e.g., smoking), use of health care services, and many other confounders that can obfuscate the relationships between the use of these medications and multiple health outcomes, including mortality. Several recent studies have begun to untangle these complex relationships and provide an initial yet complex picture of these long-term health impacts.

A large study conducted by Christoph Correll and colleagues (2015) uncovered some alarming health trends associated with the long-term use of second-generation antipsychotics. This team of investigators from the Feinstein Institute for Medical Research in Manhasset, New York, used U.S. health care claims data from 2006 to 2010, which included 284,234 adults between the ages of 18 and 65, to compare cardiovascular and cerebrovascular outcomes between people exposed to either second-generation antipsychotics or antidepressant medications. Their use of a comparison condition that was exposed to antidepressant medications is an important methodological strength of this study because both medications have similar cardiometabolic side effects and produce similar adverse CVD and cerebrovascular outcomes. These two populations of patients also share background risk factors for poor health because people with schizophrenia or depression tend to engage in similar unhealthy lifestyle behaviors. These similarities provide a clever methodological approach for controlling for common confounders related to CVD and cerebrovascular outcomes and can help isolate the impact that these medications have on these health outcomes.

Correll and colleagues (2015) found that compared to people taking antidepressants, exposure to second-generation antipsychotic medications was significantly related to higher risk for hypertension, diabetes mellitus, hypertensive heart disease, stroke, coronary artery disease, and

hyperlipidemia. These findings demonstrate that even within a short 2-year follow-up period, the use of second-generation antipsychotics was related to significant increases in the risk for both proximal and distal CVD and cerebrovascular outcomes. These results need to be replicated in other samples and populations, but they raise important concerns about the long-term physical health consequences and safety of these medications.

Newer studies using large national registries are finding a more nuanced relationship between exposures to these medications over time and long-term physical health impacts and mortality among people with SMI. Vermeulen and colleagues (2017), from the Department of Psychiatry at the Academic Medical Center in Amsterdam, have published the most comprehensive literature review and meta-analysis to date examining the link between antipsychotic medications and mortality in people with schizophrenia. They examined longitudinal data from 20 published studies with follow-up periods ranging from 1.25 to 14 years. They found a consistent trend of increased mortality risk in people with schizophrenia who did not use antipsychotic medications during the follow-up period when compared to those exposed to these medications.

Similar trends have been reported in other studies. For instance, using national registry data from Sweden, Torniainen et al. (2015) found that in a 5-year follow-up period between January 1, 2006, and December 31, 2010, the cumulative use of antipsychotic medications displayed a U-shape association with all-cause mortality (Figure 3.1). This association indicated that the highest risk of death was among people with schizophrenia with no antipsychotic use followed by high antipsychotic use. The lowest risk of death for overall mortality was observed among people at the bottom of the U-curve with low and moderate antipsychotic exposure. A similar U-shaped association was reported for CVD and cancer-related mortality and exposure to antipsychotic medications, indicating that low and moderate exposure were associated with substantially lower risk of death for these conditions than either no or high exposure (Torniainen et al., 2015).

What conclusion can we make to date regarding the long-term health impacts of antipsychotic medications given these counterintuitive findings? On the one hand, the use of these medications, particularly second-generation antipsychotics, is associated with greater risk for cardiometabolic side effects linked to serious chronic illnesses (e.g., diabetes mellitus, CVD) disproportionally impacting people with SMI. On the other hand, large national registry studies are consistently finding that long-term exposure to

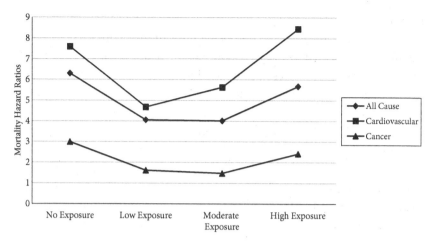

Figure 3.1 Mortality hazard ratios for adults with schizophrenia compared to the general population, stratified by levels of exposure to antipsychotic medications.

Note: Figure was orignially developed for this book presenting results reported in Torniainen et al. (2015).

antipsychotics, particularly low and moderate use, is significantly associated with lower all-cause mortality rates and deaths due to CVD or cancer compared to people with SMI not exposed to these medications. Experts in the field have concluded that given the evidence to date, there is a "favorable risk-benefit balance for the long-term use of antipsychotics in schizophrenia [and other SMIs] in reducing mortality" (Correll et al., 2018, p. 153).

The existing evidence suggests that factors beyond the use of antipsychotic medications may be more important in driving the poor health outcomes and premature mortality of people with SMI, including unhealthy behaviors; poor access, use, and quality of health and mental health services; social deprivation; illness severity; and disability. Moreover, the use of antipsychotic medications may be a proxy for better health because it suggests patients who take such medications may be better connected to health and mental health services compared to those not taking these medications. Another plausible explanation for these findings is that the use of antipsychotic medication may lead to better health behaviors because they result in improvements in psychiatric symptoms and reduce relapse. Given the state of the evidence, firm conclusions as to whether the use of antipsychotic medications is a key determinant of early mortality among people with SMI cannot be drawn at this time (Vermeulen et al., 2017). The existing studies may be uncovering

just the tip of the iceberg and providing an imperfect picture of the long-term health consequence of these medications. More work is greatly needed because second-generation antipsychotics are the mainstay treatment for SMI and their use continues to grow in this population (Correll et al., 2018).

. The associations between second-generation antipsychotic medications and their physical health side effects prompted the FDA to add warning labels about the metabolic side effects of these medications (ADA et al., 2004) to alert patients, family members, and clinicians about the potential physical health issues related to these medications. Moreover, several national and international professional associations have developed screening and monitoring guidelines for clinicians prescribing these medications. For example, one of the first guidelines was developed in 2003 via a collaboration between the ADA, the American Psychiatric Association, the American Association of Clinical Endocrinologists, and the North American Association for the Study of Obesity. These groups convened a 3-day conference in which experts from the fields of psychiatry, obesity, and diabetes as well as representatives from the FDA and pharmaceutical companies, including AstraZeneca, Bristol-Myers Squib, Janssen, Eli Lilly, and Pfizer, presented to a panel of eight members the latest research on the links between antipsychotic medications, obesity, and diabetes (ADA et al., 2004). The panel also reviewed current published evidence from epidemiological, clinical, and animal studies. These discussions and review of the literature resulted in the generation of a monitoring guideline for patients prescribed second-generation antipsychotics that focuses on tracking patients' BMI, waist circumference, blood pressure, fasting plasma glucose, and fasting lipid profile.

Newer guidelines for monitoring and managing the physical health conditions and cardiometabolic side effects of psychiatric medications in people with SMI continue to emerge. In 2009, a joint effort between the European Psychiatric Association (EPA), European Association for the Study of Diabetes (EASD), and European Society of Cardiology (ESC) resulted in the publication of cardiovascular risk management guidelines for people with SMI (De Hert et al., 2009). The goals of these guidelines are to increase the awareness and integration of services among health and mental health professionals in order to screen for, monitor, and treat cardiovascular and diabetes risk factors linked to the side effects of antipsychotic medications.

More recently, in 2018 the World Health Organization (WHO, 2018) released the *Guidelines on the Management of Physical Health*

Conditions in Adults With Severe Mental Disorders. This seminal report described up-to-date evidence-based screening, monitoring, and treatment recommendations for addressing the most pressing health conditions and cardiometabolic risk factors influencing the lives of people with SMI around the world. The goals of these guidelines were "to improve the management of physical health conditions in adults with [SMI] and support the reduction of individual health behaviors constituting risk factors for these illnesses, with the aim of decreasing morbidity and premature mortality amongst people with [SMI]" (WHO, 2018, p. 4).

Despite the publication and dissemination of these guidelines, most people with SMI taking antipsychotic medications are not routinely monitored for CVD risk factors and related health conditions in routine practice settings (De Hert, Detraux, et al., 2011), which contributes to their poor physical health. More troublesome is that many do not receive appropriate medical care when these risk factors and conditions are identified (De Hert, Cohen, et al., 2011). For instance, in the CATIE trial, 89% of participants with dyslipidemia, 62% with hypertension, and 45% with diabetes at baseline were not receiving any treatments for these conditions (Nasrallah et al., 2006). The lack of treatment was even higher for racial and ethnic minorities in this trial. Ninety-three percent of Latino/as with dyslipidemia, 79% of Latinos with hypertension, and 60% of non-White females, including Latinas, with diabetes at baseline were not receiving any treatments for these conditions (Nasrallah et al., 2006). It is important to remember that these are all adults with schizophrenia enrolled in a large clinical trial conducted in major medical centers across the United States. These rates may be an underestimation of the lack of treatment in routine practice settings that do not have the resources, expertise, and infrastructure usually available in clinical trials.

In the United States, community mental health centers are the largest front-line service setting for people with SMI in the public mental health system (Druss et al., 2008). These centers play a central role in delivering care for people with SMI. A large national survey of 181 community mental health centers found serious discrepancies in the capacity of these centers to provide basic care for the medical conditions in this population (Druss et al., 2008). Even though more than two thirds had protocols and procedures in place to screen people with SMI for common medical problems and side effects of antipsychotic medications (e.g., hypertension, obesity, diabetes), only about half reported providing treatments or referrals for these conditions. Moreover, less than a third provided general medical services for

these common medical conditions on site (Druss et al., 2008). Similarly, most children starting treatment with second-generation antipsychotics do not receive the recommended screenings for blood glucose and lipids even though they are the most vulnerable patients for developing metabolic abnormalities and for whom preventive efforts via careful screening, monitoring, and proactive early interventions can have the most benefits (De Hert, Detraux, et al., 2011).

In response to these gaps in care, multiple initiatives and programs have been developed and tested focusing on screening, monitoring for the physical health side effects of antipsychotic medications, and connecting people with SMI with the appropriate medical care to address these health conditions. Here we describe two exemplar programs that aim to improve the health and wellness of people with SMI by integrating health and mental health services and improving the screening, monitoring, and treatment of the common cardiometabolic side effects of antipsychotic medications. These two examples by no means represent all the interventions and programs that currently exist to address these critical health and health care inequities in people with SMI. The reason for describing these two programs is that they illustrate two different approaches to tackling these health care inequities. One focuses on improving the integration of primary care services in behavioral health organizations to improve the access, use, and quality of health care for adults with SMI. This program intends to bring primary care to the settings where most people with SMI receive care. The other takes a preventive approach by focusing on preventing antipsychotic-induced weight gain among people experiencing their first psychotic episode and taking antipsychotic medications. In this approach, the emphasis is on targeting physical health issues before they turn into chronic medical issues, and it treats physical health as an important component of mental health treatments from the very beginning of care.

In 2009, the U.S. Substance Abuse and Mental Health Service Administration (SAMHSA) launched a large-scale initiative called the Primary and Behavioral Health Care Integration (PBHCI) program (Scharf et al., 2013). This program is now led by the National Council for Mental Wellbeing (2020) at their Center of Excellence for Integrated Health Solutions. The PBHCI's goal was to improve the wellness and physical health of adults with SMI by developing service infrastructures to support the availability, coordination, delivery, and integration of primary care services in community mental health centers or other community-based behavioral

health organizations. In this national program, behavioral health organizations received up to half a million dollars per year for 4 years to develop integrated services that included four key features: screening and referral for physical health care, tracking system for people's physical health needs and outcomes, care management services, and prevention and wellness services. As of 2016, more than 200 grants have been awarded throughout the continental United States, Hawaii, and Alaska.

In 2013, the RAND Corporation published findings from an initial evaluation of the PBHCI program (Scharf et al., 2013). Part of this evaluation was to examine whether people with SMI enrolled in PBHCI programs showed improvements in health and mental health outcomes. To answer this important question, the RAND team used a quasi-experimental design to compare clients' health and mental health outcomes over a 12-month period between three PBHCI sites and three matched control sites not participating in the PBHCI program. Results showed that compared to clients in the matched sites, the PBHCI clients reported statistically significant reductions in diastolic blood pressure, total cholesterol, low-density lipoprotein cholesterol, and fasting plasma glucose. No significant differences between sites were observed for systolic blood pressure, BMI, high-density lipoprotein cholesterol, glycated hemoglobin, triglycerides, self-reported smoking, and behavioral health outcomes (e.g., self-reported social connectedness, perceived health; Scharf et al., 2013). These initial findings are promising and suggest that for people with SMI, programs like the PBHCI can produce important health benefits and connect them to needed medical care. More work is needed to strengthen the quality of care delivered by these types of programs and to increase their accessibility and impact in the community.

The second program takes a preventive approach and focuses on averting antipsychotic-induced weight gain in people experiencing their first episode of psychosis (FEP). The program was developed by Jackie Curtis and colleagues from the Early Psychosis Program at the Bondi Center in Sydney, Australia, and from the School of Psychiatry at the University of New South Wales. The program, Keeping the Body in Mind (KBIM), was described in a pilot study published in the journal *Early Intervention in Psychiatry* (Curtis et al., 2016). I also had an opportunity to interview Dr. Curtis about KBIM and her work in April 2019, as we were both attending and presenting at the Schizophrenia International Research Society conference, which was being held that year in Orlando, Florida.

According to Dr. Kurtis, KBIM arose from her own clinical work as she was seeing her patients with FEP putting on weight right in front of her eyes over a matter of weeks, particularly those on olanzapine. She described how her patients "put on 10, 20, 30 kilograms, translate that into pounds, its massive. I see this within 3 or 4 weeks." She observed this weight gain back in 2002 when there were no clinical guidelines on how to best counteract it among people with FEP taking second-generation antipsychotic medications. She and her team began this work by measuring and monitoring their patients' weight, height, blood pressure, and other metabolic indicators (e.g., blood glucose, lipids), which she based on the work that Dr. David Henderson from Boston was doing examining the links between diabetes and psychosis. In short, they created their own protocol to monitor the health of their patients.

By tracking these basic health indicators, her team began to see how their patients' health was deteriorating. They soon realized they had found a problem that needed an intervention. This realization prompted them to train their nurses on diabetes prevention and treatment and to bring other health specialists (e.g., dieticians, exercise physiologists) into their clinical team who had expertise in healthy lifestyle changes. They also realized that they needed to do something at their clinic rather than just send their patients to primary care because many of the general practitioners in primary care were not trained to address the physical health of young people with FEP.

To address this growing need, Dr. Curtis talked to me about developing "a robust response. . . . Don't just screen, intervene." KBIM arose organically in small incremental steps shaped by the central principle of taking care of the patient's whole body, not just their minds. They wanted the program to be practical, attractive to young people, socially interactive, and integrated into their FEP services. Their goal was to introduce healthy lifestyles right from the very beginning: "rather than waiting for the risk factors to accumulate, right from the start check on all risk factors, so smoking, diet, activity, weight, blood pressure, glucose, and so on. And then straightaway, lifestyle advice to include diet, physical activity, and smoking prevention or cessation," she told me.

Today, KBIM has matured into an individualized healthy lifestyle and life skills intervention for youth with FEP who are initiating treatment with antipsychotic medications. The intervention is delivered in specialized FEP clinics by a team of clinicians, including a clinical nurse consultant, dietician, exercise physiologist, and two youth peer wellness coaches who are young

people with lived experiences coping with antipsychotic-induced weight gain. A psychiatrist and endocrinologist provided additional support to this team.

KBIM comprises three interrelated components. The first is health coaching to maximize motivation and increase participation. The second is dietetic support via weekly visits with a dietician to support healthy eating, weight management, delivery of educational modules around food quality, portion control, reading and understanding nutritional labels, and cooking skills, among other topics. This support also helped participants learn how to prepare healthy meals and shop for healthy foods. The third component focuses on physical activity. An exercise physiologist worked with each participant to develop an individualized exercise program based on participants' fitness level, motivation, goals, and psychiatric needs. The goal was for participants to engage in regular physical activity. To support engagement in regular exercise, participants had access to and were encouraged to use the supervised gym available at their FEP clinic, which included treadmills, stationary bikes, and resistance training equipment. Two other important elements of KBIM were the youth peer wellness coaches and antipsychotic medication switching. Peer wellness coaches served as role models to provide motivation and encouragement to keep participants engaged in the intervention. Medical staff also closely monitored participants' weight gain and switched medications in any participant who gained more than 5 kg (11 lb) to a more weight-neutral antipsychotic medication.

In a small pilot study comparing KBIM ($n = 26$) to usual FEP care ($n = 23$), Curtis and colleagues (2016) found that KBIM participants, particularly those who completed the program, experienced significantly less weight gain at 12 weeks compared to participants receiving usual FEP care. Moreover, a lower proportion of KBIM participants experienced clinically significant weight gain (greater than 7% of baseline weight) than those in the usual care group, 13% vs. 75%, respectively. These results are promising and suggest that an individualized program like KBIM integrated into standard FEP services can help attenuate antipsychotic-induced weight gain among people initiating treatment with these medications.

KBIM is now being offered in multiple community mental health centers in Australia specializing in FEP. Reflecting upon this great work, Dr. Curtis told me she attributed the success of KBIM to the idea that the "physical health element just feels much more normalizing to someone. I don't know what it is; I think it also brings a routine. It also feels like some sense of

personal control and self-efficacy that I don't think . . . all our interventions do that. So, I think it's been surprisingly popular. We observed the problem. We quantified the problem. And then we tried to work out an intervention."

More work is greatly needed to rigorously examine the effectiveness of these preventive efforts and, if shown to be effective, how to best integrate them into routine practice settings. The focus on health prevention and promotion is gaining support and attention from mental health professionals, medical doctors, advocates, researchers, family members, and people living with SMI. A great example of this renewed interest in health promotion for people with SMI is the Healthy Active Lives (HeAL) initiative developed by a group of clinicians, service users, family members, and researchers from 11 countries. This group produced a consensus and aspirational statement that set forward a set of practice values, standards, and guidelines aiming to "reverse the trend of people with severe mental illness dying early by tackling risks for future physical illnesses pro-actively and much earlier" (iphYs, 2018). A health prevention perspective and practice are important for people with SMI because they may help "prevent the seeding of future disease risk and in the long-term help reduce the life expectancy gap for people living with SMI" (Curtis et al., 2016, p. 1).

4

"They Do Not Get the Care That They Need"

Martin Luther King Jr. described inequities in health care as the most shocking and inhumane injustices in our society (Dittmer, 2009). These injustices are unfair differences between populations in their access to, use of, quality of, and outcomes of health care driven not by needs or preferences but by people's backgrounds (Institute of Medicine, 2003). Inequities arise when people do not receive appropriate health care because of the color of their skin, where they live, whether they have health insurance, the language they speak, and other personal factors. In an equitable health care system, none of these personal characteristics should prevent anyone from accessing or receiving the health care they need. For people with serious mental illness (SMI), these injustices in health care are common and can be deadly. What makes inequities in health care so shocking, in my opinion, is that they occur because the providers, organizations, and communities responsible for delivering care fail to do their jobs, resulting in avoidable suffering, pain, and in some instances death (Cabassa, 2016). For many people with SMI, as we will see in this chapter, their experiences with the health care system are indeed unjust, shocking, and dehumanizing, exacerbating their health problems and contributing to premature mortality. Cristina's health care experiences are a case in point.

Cristina was in her mid-60s when she told us how she came to be diagnosed and treated for cancer. She came to our attention as part of a study we were conducting to learn about the health care experiences of Latino/as with SMI. Part of her story is described in an article we published in 2014 (Cabassa, Gomes, Meyreles, Capitelli, Younge, Dragatsi, Alvarez, Nicasio et al., 2014). When we met, she was in remission, but her struggles to get medical care were still fresh in her mind.

Cristina is barely 5 feet tall. She looks like a typical grandmother, with short white hair, and deep wrinkles throughout her face. She is soft-spoken and looks a bit fragile; she loves to tell stories and always greets you with

Addressing Health Inequities in People With Serious Mental Illness. Leopoldo J. Cabassa, Oxford University Press.
© Oxford University Press 2023. DOI: 10.1093/oso/9780190937300.003.0004

a heartwarming smile that lights up her entire face. Cristina was born in New York City. Her parents, both Cuban, immigrated to New York in the late 1940s. She is fluent in both English and Spanish and never married. Cristina has worked odd jobs since she was 16 years old to help her family make ends meet and did not finish high school. In her mid-20s, she was hospitalized after a serious psychotic episode, which involved a suicide attempt. She was diagnosed with schizoaffective disorder and since then has been under outpatient psychiatric care. At the time of our study, she was a long-time patient of a public outpatient mental health clinic and was well known and loved by the clinic's staff.

In her early 40s, she was diagnosed with diabetes and high cholesterol and began taking medications for these conditions. Shortly after, she began to experience what she described as "strange physical symptoms." She started having sharp pains in her lower abdomen and felt tired all the time. Concerned about these symptoms, she went to her primary care doctor, who recommended she go to the emergency room (ER). That is when things went south for Cristina.

Cristina described how the doctors and nurses in the ER doubted that her physical pain and symptoms were real. No matter how much she complained and pleaded with the medical staff, they focused on her schizoaffective disorder and the psychiatric medications (i.e., olanzapine) she was taking at that time. They even called for a psychiatric consult given her history of psychiatric hospitalizations. She ended up hospitalized, not in a medical unit, but in the psychiatric ward. She mentioned how the doctors at that time told her "everything is fine, and they stick me in psychiatry. They don't pay attention. I can go with a pain, and they commit me—instead of admitting me to the hospital to check me" (as qtd. in Cabassa, Gomes, Meyreles, Capitelli, Younge, Dragatsi, Alvarez, Nicasio et al., 2014, p. 731).

She was in the psychiatric unit for 3 weeks. During this time, her symptoms worsened, her pain intensified, yet she was provided little relief or treatments for her pain. The medical staff continued to consider her symptoms and complaints as part of her mental illness, not a physical medical condition. It got so bad that she started to urinate blood. At that point the medical staff realized something was seriously wrong with Cristina and that her physical symptoms and complaints were not in her head but were in fact a medical condition that required medical intervention. Cristina described how it was then "when they discovered that I had cancer" (as qtd. in Cabassa, Gomes, Meyreles, Capitelli, Younge, Dragatsi, Alvarez, Nicasio et al., 2014, p. 731).

They finally transferred her to a medical unit and operated on her. It took this ordeal for Cristina to receive medical care for her cancer.

Sadly, Cristina's struggles to receive timely medical care are common. Like Cristina, people with SMI experience persistent inequities in accessing, using, and receiving high-quality health care. Along with the factors described in the previous chapters, unhealthy lifestyle behaviors in unhealthy environments and the cardiometabolic side effects of antipsychotic medications, these inequities in health care also contribute to the poor physical health outcomes and premature mortality experienced by people with SMI. These inequities exist along the entire continuum of care, from accessing health care services and receiving appropriate screening and preventive care to being properly diagnosed and treated for common chronic medical illnesses.

Access is fundamental to health care, yet people with SMI tend to face multiple barriers accessing and receiving medical care even when they have public or private health insurance. For example, Bradford and colleagues (2008) in an article published in the journal *Psychiatric Services* compared access and barriers to medical care among people with and without SMI. They used data from the National Health Interview Survey, a nationally representative study sponsored by the U.S. Centers for Disease Control and Prevention (CDC) that examines health-related issues in the U.S. noninstitutionalized population. They found that among 156,475 adults over the age of 18, people with psychotic or bipolar disorders had significantly lower odds of having a regular source of primary medical care than people without these disorders. Moreover, people with psychotic, bipolar, or major depressive disorders consistently reported significantly higher odds compared to people without these disorders in being unable to get medical care in times of need, delaying medical care because of cost concerns, and being unable to get needed prescription medications. Each of these findings held even after adjusting for differences in age, sex, race, education, income, health insurance, and the presence of alcohol or drug use disorders between people with and without SMI.

Even when people with SMI access medical services, the quality of care they receive may be poor. People with SMI face large deficits in the quality of care they receive for preventive services, cardiovascular disease, diabetes, cancer screenings and treatments, and other medical conditions (De Hert, Cohen et al., 2011; Mangurian et al., 2016; McGinty et al., 2015b). These gaps in the quality of medical care vary substantially depending on the settings of

care being studied (e.g., public or private hospitals, Veterans Administration [VA] facilities, outpatient clinics), the medical conditions being examined, and the methods used to study these gaps (McGinty et al., 2015b; Mitchell & Lord, 2010). For example, in a large retrospective cohort study using data from the California Medicaid program, Mangurian and colleagues (2015) found that among 50,915 adults 18 years of age or older with an SMI diagnosis and receiving a prescription for an antipsychotic medication, only 30.1% had received the recommended screening for diabetes mellitus using validated measures (e.g., glucose-specific fasting serum, glycated hemoglobin test). This finding illustrates how in one of the largest public mental health systems in the United States, almost 70% of adults with SMI receiving an antipsychotic medication did not receive the recommended screenings for diabetes mellitus.

Consistent with the low rates of screening for diabetes and cardiovascular risk factors, people with SMI also tend to not receive timely screening for breast, cervical, prostate, and colorectal cancers (Weinstein et al., 2016). For instance, in a series of studies using a retrospective population-based design examining health records in the Canadian province of Manitoba, women with schizophrenia were approximately 30% less likely to receive a cervical cancer screening and almost 40% less likely to have a mammography (Chochinov et al., 2009; Martens et al., 2009). In a more recent systematic literature review led by Dr. Lara Weinstein from Thomas Jefferson University in Philadelphia, her team concluded that most studies show lower rates of cancer screening in people with schizophrenia or psychosis compared to people without these mental disorders, even in health care systems that provide free access to screening services (Weinstein et al., 2016).

These deficits in the medical care for people SMI are also costly. Christina Mangurian and colleagues from the University of California in San Francisco, using data from a literature review on diabetes and cardiovascular care for people with SMI, provided sobering statistics for these preventable health care costs (Mangurian et al., 2016). They estimated that because 20% of the 19 million adults with SMI in the United States have diabetes and about 70% of them are not properly screened, it is plausible that over 2 million people with SMI in the United States have unidentified diabetes and other cardiovascular diseases. Moreover, since undiagnosed diabetes costs approximately $4,000 per person, these deficits in care for people with SMI may result in over $8 billion in annual costs to our health care system. All these costs can be prevented with appropriate screening, monitoring, and treatment. Yet

more than a decade since the publication of numerous treatment guidelines for people with SMI, these costs continue to persist and grow.

A key question that requires careful attention is, do gaps in the quality of medical care contribute to premature mortality in people with SMI? The answers to this important question are mixed. There is evidence to suggest that for some conditions and medical procedures it does (Druss et al., 2001); however, others have not found that the difference in quality of medical care directly contributes to premature mortality in people with SMI (McGinty et al., 2012). More research is needed to examine this important question across the major medical conditions (e.g., cardiovascular disease, diabetes, cancer) related to premature mortality in people with SMI.

One of the most cited studies examining the relationship between quality of medical care and premature mortality among people with SMI was published by Benjamin Druss and colleagues (2001) from Emory University. They analyzed data from a cohort of 88,241 Medicare patients 65 years and older to investigate the association between mental disorders (e.g., schizophrenia, affective disorders), quality of medical care, and mortality in the first year after a myocardial infraction. They found that after adjusting for a variety of factors associated with death after a myocardial infraction (e.g., age, race, cardiac history, socioeconomic status), people with a mental disorder had a 19% increased likelihood of dying during the year after being discharged from the hospital compared to people without mental disorders. A similar pattern of elevated risk of death was observed for people with specific mental disorders: 34% increased likelihood for people with schizophrenia and 11% increased likelihood for people with affective disorders.

After adjusting for all covariates and five established quality-of-care indicators after a myocardial infarction (e.g., reperfusion, aspirin, β-blockers, angiotensin-converting enzyme [ACE] inhibitors, smoking cessation counseling), the association between mortality and mental disorders was no longer significant, and overall mortality reduced by 9%, almost half of the original value of excess mortality (Druss et al., 2001). A similar pattern was observed for each of the mental disorders examined in this study. These findings revealed that the differences in mortality rates between people with and without mental disorders in this study seemed to have been accounted for in part by differences in the quality of medical care these groups of people received after a myocardial infarction. Overall, the findings from Druss et al.'s

(2001) study illustrate that deficits in the quality of medical care can, in some instances, explain a substantial portion of the excess mortality experienced by people with SMI, particularly after a myocardial infarction.

Despite the mixed results examining the relationships between quality of medical care and premature mortality among people with SMI, it is evident that the health care system frequently fails to provide people with SMI high-quality care for medical conditions. Numerous government reports and literature reviews have consistently concluded that a constellation of system-, provider-, interpersonal-, and patient-level factors contribute to health care inequities in people with SMI (Firth et al., 2019; Institute of Medicine, 2006; Liu et al., 2017; McGinty et al., 2015b). It is beyond the scope of this book to describe all these factors and how they interact to create inequities in health care for people with SMI. Here, I would like to illustrate some of the factors we have found in our work to be critical in shaping the health care of people with SMI. The factors highlighted are also modifiable, meaning they can be targets for intervention and inform the development of programs designed to help reduce these inequities in health care.

Over the years, my team and I have conducted numerous interviews and focus group discussions with psychiatrists, social workers, nurses, primary care physicians, directors and administrators of clinics, community leaders, people living with SMI and their family members, and researchers. These multiple perspectives provided us with a deep understanding of the interplay of factors (e.g., system-level barriers, stigma and discrimination, mistrust) that shape the health care experiences of people with SMI. One of the best descriptions of these interactions came from an administrator of a public mental health clinic in New York City. In fact, the title of this chapter comes from her description. She described the challenges that her patients with SMI, particularly her Latino/a patients, faced when navigating the health care system in this way. "I think that our patients, partly because of their illnesses . . . partly because of the cultural and language issues, and partly because the system is not very well organized—they often get lost in the system. . . . The patients just get overwhelmed. . . . [Y]ou imagine, you're not feeling well, you may have symptoms of psychosis; you don't speak the language, and you're trying to figure out what office to go to; it can be overwhelming, and patients get frustrated and don't get the care that they need" (Ezell et al., 2013, p. 1560).

Fragmented Health Care System

The poor quality of health care that people with SMI receive is often a result of the configuration and organization of our health care system, a system that has historically tended to separate health care and mental health care from each other structurally, administratively, financially, legally, and in many instances physically (Institute of Medicine, 2006). The separation between our mental health care and general health care systems is so big that it has been characterized as a "chasm" (Hogan, 2003). This separation creates serious difficulties for everyone involved in caring for people with SMI because it requires people to navigate through what often feels like a never-ending labyrinth of bureaucracies, paperwork, and multiple locations, and to do so within systems of care that frequently do not communicate and collaborate with or trust each other. It is left to the patient, their family members, and their providers to find their way through these complex systems of care, which often results in people falling through the cracks and not getting the health care they deserve and need.

The most common complaint we hear from people with SMI and everyone involved in their care is that our entire system of care is broken, even for those who have private or public health insurance. In a series of focus group discussions we conducted with Latino/a patients with SMI about their experiences using primary health care services in their urban communities, all described having to navigate and interact with a stressed health care system (Cabassa, Gomes, Meyreles, Capitelli, Younge, Dragatsi, Alvarez, Nicasio et al., 2014). All our participants consistently talked about how their primary care clinics were always overflowing with patients, and that the staff—from the receptionists to the doctors—were overburdened and rushed. Another common experience was having to wait for months to get an appointment, which frustrated many of our participants given their complex and chronic medical conditions. Other common barriers we documented include having to wait for hours to see a doctor in cramped and noisy waiting rooms and not being able to form lasting relationships with health care providers due to high staff turnover and overreliance at many clinics to use health care providers in training. Each of these system-level barriers tended to erode people's confidence and trust in the health care system, and for many, it pushed them to delay or avoid medical care.

Stigma and Discrimination

Beyond these system-level obstacles, stigma and discrimination are persistent barriers to medical care among historically marginalized and underserved populations (Institute of Medicine, 2003). Multiple studies have shown how people with SMI are often discriminated against by health care providers, resulting in people avoiding and disengaging from medical care (Borba et al., 2012; Thornicroft, 2006). In our own work, we have seen how stigma, racism, and discrimination are common experiences for people with SMI, particularly from brown and Black communities, negatively affecting their interactions with the health care system. In a survey we conducted with 40 Latino/a adults with SMI at a public mental health clinic, 75% reported that racism was a problem in the U.S. health care system (Cabassa, Gomes, Meyreles, Capitelli, Younge, Dragatsi, Alvarez, Nicasio et al., 2014). Moreover, the majority of participants in this survey also reported that people are treated unjustly in the health care system not only because of their mental illness but also because of the combination of other social identities historically marginalized in the United States, such as being a member of an ethnic group, being an immigrant, being Black, or speaking Spanish as their primary language. What is telling about the findings from this small convenience sample of Latino/a participants was that they had health insurance (e.g., Medicaid) and had access to primary care services. All but one had visited a primary care clinic in the past year, so these findings reflect what they see, feel, and experience as they use these services. These findings by no means are representative of all people with SMI, but they do provide a window into how some people with SMI who use primary care services are treated in segments of our health care system.

The combination of stigma toward mental illness and racism can result in discrimination within the medical encounter that negatively affects the quality and outcomes of medical care for people with SMI. As we and others have discussed, labeling a person with a psychiatric condition can result in a phenomenon known as *diagnostic overshadowing*, in which the label of mental illness activates multiple biases among providers to the point where they question, doubt, and even ignore the person's medical complaints and incorrectly assume they are part of the person's mental illness (Jones et al., 2008). This neglect often results is misdiagnoses and in recommending

the wrong treatment or even withholding treatment. Cristina's experience described earlier in this chapter is an illustration of this common phenomenon.

In our work, we described how on top of diagnostic overshadowing, a person's racial and ethnic minoritized status can activate other biases, such as concluding that the person's physical complaints are the somatization of psychological symptoms (e.g., headaches due to stress, stomach pain due to anxiety) rather than true signs of a physical illness (Cabassa, Siantz, et al. 2014). This phenomenon is common for Latino/a patients, and similar to diagnostic overshadowing, it can result in misdiagnosis and not receiving appropriate medical care (Escobar et al., 1987). Both of these biases can be compounded by cultural and linguistic differences between providers and patients, the multiple demands and pressures that clinicians face in busy and under-resourced and understaffed clinics, the limited time that providers have to see patients and make diagnostic and treatment decisions, and the lack of familiarity providers may have with patients' complex medical history (Cabassa, Siantz, et al., 2014). Isabel's and Angela's experiences seeking medical care, which we described in a previous paper, illustrate how the interactions of stigma and racism can shape the health care experiences of people with SMI (Cabassa, Gomes, Meyreles, Capitelli, Younge, Dragatsi, Alvarez, Nicasio et al., 2014).

Isabel, a Cuban immigrant in her mid-50s who was enrolled in one of our studies, described a negative interaction she had while seeking care for her asthma. At the time of this event she was diagnosed with a schizoaffective disorder, hypertension, and asthma. We detailed her case in an article published in *Administration and Policy in Mental Health and Mental Health Services Research*:

Isabel recounted how she experienced discrimination seeking medical attention for respiratory problems and chest pains. Isabel arrived at her clinic accompanied by her brother and asked to see her doctor even though she did not have an appointment. The receptionist wrote down her name, and she waited to be seen. After two hours of worsening symptoms, Isabel approached a staff nurse to find out how much longer it would be and stressed that she was having trouble breathing. The nurse informed her that she could not be seen that day as she did not have an appointment. At that point, Isabel recounts that she became irate [and] explained that her name had already been taken down by the receptionist two hours ago.

She stated she wanted to be seen by a doctor as it was an emergency, and she had been a patient at the clinic for 15 years. According to Isabel, the staff member replied, "You Hispanics are always sick. You never get well." At this point, Isabel began arguing with the nurse and, in response to her racist remark, told the nurse, "It is because of us Hispanics that you eat in your home . . . that you pay your rent. . . . And let me tell you something, you're not a professional, because a professional would not speak to a patient the way you are speaking to me." (Cabassa Meyreles, Capitelli, Younge, Dragatsi, Alvarez, Nicasio et al., 2014, p. 731)

After another nurse at the clinic got involved, Isabel and her brother were finally taken to an examination room. They remained in the examination room for another hour while her symptoms continued, until her brother lost his patience and pleaded with the staff to provide medical attention to his sister. When the doctor finally came into the room, he told Isabel that he had forgotten that she was in there, which only upset and offended her further. Isabel recounted that she ended her appointment crying out of anger, frustration, and physical discomfort. When asked during the focus group about this experience, she replied, "A person becomes depressed. I started to cry. I wanted to die from crying. I asked myself, 'What is this?'" (Cabassa, Gomes, Meyreles, Capitelli, Younge, Dragatsi, Alvarez, Nicasio et al., 2014, p. 731)

Isabel's experience illustrates the treatment some people with SMI receive from the health care system. The combination of stigma and discrimination within the medical encounter is extremely detrimental because it makes people feel dehumanized and disrespected by the system of care whose purpose and mission are to help them during times of need and vulnerability.

Angela was in her 40s when she described the following experience in a focus group we conducted at an outpatient mental health clinic. To this day, I can still remember how angry, frustrated, and sad she was describing how she was treated, even though this had occurred several years ago. Angela was born in Mexico, never finished high school, and had lived in New York City for more than a decade. She spoke mostly Spanish. At the time of our study, she was diagnosed with major depression, generalized anxiety disorder, hypertension, arthritis, diabetes, high cholesterol, and asthma. She lived by herself but had several family members living nearby. She described being close with her siblings, cousins, and other extended family members. When we

asked the group to describe any negative experiences that they had seeking medical care, Angela related the following situation.

> I had a White doctor for about 5–7 years, and I came to understand that she made grave mistakes. For example, I fell and ripped two tendons [while at work], a bone came out of place, and I had a lot of arthritis here. . . . And I waited one year for her to pay attention to me because I went to her immediately when I fell. I told her I had a lot of pain and she told me, "Go to [physical] therapy and take an anti-anxiety pill." . . . Exactly one year passed. And I couldn't handle the pain anymore. I would go to the [physical] therapies. That did nothing for me. And I changed therapists. And when I changed therapists, changed clinics . . . I said to my new [Hispanic] doctor, "Since I take pills for depression, tell me if it's that I'm going crazy or if it's that I have something, because I have a pain here that I can't take and my [previous] doctor doesn't pay attention to me." So that's when she took action, but it took a year. They did tests and it came out that I had a problem. They did an MRI and it showed that I had two ripped tendons. All of that could have been avoided. I lost my job. I lost my apartment. I lost everything because they had to operate on me. (Cabassa, Gomes, Meyreles, Capitelli, Younge, Dragatsi, Alvarez, Nicasio et al., 2014, p. 732)

Angela's experience also touches upon a critical reality that is often not openly discussed about the health care inequities experienced by people with SMI. Her example illustrates how serious lapses in medical care not only negatively affected her physical and emotional health but also threatened her livelihood. Angela's case depicts the interconnection between health care and multiple social determinants of health. Not receiving appropriate medical care can create negative ripples in a person's life, destroying their ability to work, earn a living, and pay rent. All shape a person's overall health and quality of life.

Mistrust

Mistrust of the health care system is a common reaction for people with SMI who have experienced stigma, racism, and discrimination while seeking medical care. This breakdown in trust can have multiple negative consequences for people with SMI. It can result in unnecessary delays in

care as a person may think twice before going to the doctor if they do not expect to receive appropriate treatment or to be treated fairly with dignity and respect. For people who do seek care, mistrust can result in their refusal of treatments, dropping out prematurely, or not completing recommended treatments.

We have observed in our studies how mistrust can erode the doctor–patient relationship. Establishing and maintaining trusting working relationships between patients and their medical providers is essential, particularly for people living and coping with chronic medical illnesses (e.g., diabetes, hypertension) and SMI. Treating these conditions requires a multitude of disease management activities. For example, a person will make multiple visits to their primary care provider and different medical specialists throughout the year. These visits will often require regular laboratory testing (e.g., fasting glucose, lipid panels) to monitor multiple health indicators, which will help the doctor and the patient make treatment decisions. Most often, the patient will also have to follow medication regimens involving taking multiple medications throughout the day and in different schedules (e.g., once, twice, or multiple times a day, with or without meals). Moreover, treatment will require that the person make healthy lifestyle changes to their diets and physical activity level, as well as reducing their consumption of drug and alcohol, and quitting or reducing smoking for those who smoke. And let's not forget, these are people with SMI, who on top of these chronic disease management activities must also manage and cope with the symptoms and treatments related to their mental illness. It is an understatement to say that managing all of this on a day-to-day basis is complex. If you add to this complexity the element that you do not trust the providers who are there to help you, then the tasks of managing and living with these conditions become almost insurmountable and your risk for experiencing negative health outcomes increases at an alarming rate.

Mistrusting medical providers can negatively impact the quality of medical care people with SMI receive in numerous ways. Here are two common examples from our work. First, mistrust can result in restricting patients' willingness to question doctors' advice about their medical treatment or to ask questions to clarify any doubts they may have during the medical encounter to avoid the potential of mistreatment and negative judgment. This kind of situation was best expressed by Lydia (a Black participant with schizophrenia, diabetes, and hypertension) when we asked a focus group she was participating in whether people would disagree with or question their primary care doctor: She responded:

I feel like it would be a waste of time. A lot of doctors are headstrong and they feel like they are the smartest people in the world anyways. I personally wouldn't do it. I have seen how some of the doctors act, and if you don't agree with some of the stuff then they will start mistreating you. (Cabassa, Siantz, et al., 2014, p. 1130)

Mistrust can also elevate the levels of suspicion people with SMI have when they visit their primary care doctors. It can result in people entering a medical encounter in a defensive stance, as described by Martin, a Black participant who was diagnosed with schizoaffective disorder and diabetes. During our interview, Martin described a negative encounter with his primary care doctor: "I've been to doctors like that. They don't really care about your health at all. . . . I get what I need to get from them and that's it. You don't disrespect me, I won't disrespect you. I out-fox the fox!" (as qtd. in Cabassa, Siantz, et al., 2014, p. 1130).

This defensive stance is contrary to what providers expect from their patients, and it is detrimental to the patient–provider relationship. Primary care providers are trained, at a minimum, that their patients will be willing to share and disclose their symptoms and to ask questions. Of course, some patients are better than others at communicating what they are experiencing, and it is the job of the provider to ask questions and probe to get the information they need to arrive at a potential diagnosis to inform a treatment plan. Mistrust throws a wrench into these assumptions and creates serious obstacles in the medical encounter by restricting the information that should flow between patients and their providers. A defensive, suspicious stance from patients as they enter the medical encounter is the opposite of what is needed to have a trusting working relationship with a medical provider.

The importance of trust to the patient–provider relationship is evident in the descriptions we heard from people with SMI who reported positive experiences with their primary care providers. These interactions are often described as warm, friendly, respectful, professional, and genuine. When trusting relationships exist between patients and their providers, patients feel heard and cared for. They feel supported and report that their doctor is acting in good faith and has their best interest in mind when making treatment decisions. A good example of this trusting relationship came from Gonzalo, a Puerto Rican participant with depression and high cholesterol, who talked about his primary care doctor in the following manner:

Well, I have a doctor who is *un amor* [a dear], like my grandmother says. He gives me my medications—they are for blood pressure. But he hasn't given me any more medications. In other words, instead of him telling me "this medication would be good for you," he'll more readily say, "better to eat this soup or drink this." Now, it's not that he avoids medication, but instead of prescribing me more medications he tries to tell me, "do more exercise. Eat healthier. Do this." He talks to me too. He's a good person. . . . He's a good person in that first he counsels you before you get an illness. . . . He works on prevention." (as qtd. in Cabassa, Gomes, Meyreles, Capitelli, Younge, Dragatsi, Alvarez, Nicasio et al., 2014, p. 732)

Positive relationships with providers not only are critical for receiving good-quality care but also help combat the stigma people with SMI face when interacting with the medical system. They humanize the interaction, as captured by Gonzalo's comment:

I prefer a doctor who treats me like a friend, like a person who goes there with problems, but who says . . . you know, not a person who looks at you as having a defect. Because there are people who you tell, "I have this mental or physical problem," and at once they put up a barrier. I prefer that communication occurs between the two and that he learns about my personal things. For example, "Are you married? Do you have a girlfriend?" All of those personal things my doctor knows about me. And it seems like a good thing to me, because like that he knows about me. (as qtd. in Cabassa, Gomes, Meyreles, Capitelli, Younge, Dragatsi, Alvarez, Nicasio et al., 2014, p. 733)

Positive patient–provider relationships are a critical ingredient for reducing mistrust and stigma in people with SMI. In our work we have also found that among Latino/as with SMI, having a positive relationship with their primary care doctors that reflects core cultural norms of *respeto* (respect), *dignidad* (dignity), and *persnalismo* (being warm and personable) was associated with being more satisfied with the medical care they receive, feeling more confident about their ability to manage and cope with their chronic medical illnesses, and being more involved and active in their own medical care (Cabassa, Gomes, Meyreles, Capitelli, Younge, Dragatsi, Alvarez, Nicasio et al., 2014). Cultivating positive patient–provider relationships that reflect warmth, trust, respect, dignity, and open communication could be a plausible avenue for combating stigma, discrimination, and mistrust, thus

improving the quality of medical care for people with SMI (Cabassa, Gomes, Meyreles, Capitelli, Younge, Dragatsi, Alvarez, Nicasio et al., 2014).

Professional Boundaries

Another common barrier we have observed that impacts the health care that people with SMI receive concerns what has been classified as issues with professional boundaries (Ezell et al., 2013; Kilbourne et al., 2012). These are questions and doubts regarding who is responsible and in charge of the physical health of people with SMI. In other words, whose job is it to screen, monitor, manage, and treat the medical conditions that afflict people with SMI? This uncertainty regarding providers' roles and responsibilities can result in serious deficiencies in the medical care that people with SMI receive in terms of not receiving timely screenings, diagnoses, and appropriate referrals; breakdowns in the coordination and communication between medical and mental health providers; and unnecessary delays in receiving appropriate treatments. We have found this ambivalence is more pronounced among mental health providers (e.g., social workers, psychiatrists, psychiatric nurses), who may feel that the physical health of their patients with SMI is beyond their professional duties. An administrator of a mental health clinic described this problem in an interview we conducted with them.

> I would have to say that the therapists probably are not as good at following up on these issues [referring to patients' physical health] in part because it's not their area of expertise, and they don't consider that necessarily their responsibility to worry about the patient's medical health. . . . I can't say that all of my clinicians call the patient's primary care doctor if there are health concerns. I would be shocked if they were doing that on a regular basis. (Ezell et al., 2013, p. 1562)

Lack of training, supervision, and education in the prevention and management of chronic medical illnesses, even among psychiatrists, directly contributes to these professional boundary issues, as captured by a psychiatrist we interviewed at a community mental health center: "But I'm not really monitoring them [patients with SMI] because I'm not up to date with the latest, you know, antihypertensives and the best regimen for diabetes. I want

them to get the best care possible, so I try to refer them out" (Cabassa, Siantz, et al., 2014, p. 1130).

Professional boundary issues continue to persist, even though, as we discuss in Chapter 3, numerous monitoring and treatment guidelines are available for mental health providers to address the most common cardiometabolic conditions afflicting people with SMI. Yet, these guidelines are not widely used in mental health settings.

However, professional ambivalence can disappear at times. We observed that for certain acute and life-threatening conditions, some mental health providers put aside their professional boundary concerns and intervene. A comment from a psychiatrist at an outpatient clinic exemplifies this situation. Her team got involved in addressing a pressing need impacting one of their patients:

> I think the milder cases . . . we probably need to do a better job. But the serious cases, we really work hard to help. A great example is . . . four or five years ago, one of our patients [with psychosis] needed a heart transplant, and he was very low on the list because he was psychotic, and we really advocated for him. (as qtd. in Cabassa, Siantz, et al., 2014, p. 1131)

This case highlights the need to shift the tipping point of action for mental health providers from acute to chronic care. As we have seen, people with SMI face numerous chronic medical conditions that require ongoing support and management. Mental health providers, from psychiatrists to social workers, need training, supervision, and support to clarify professional responsibilities and define their roles in screening, monitoring, managing, coordinating, and treating the most prevalent health conditions in people with SMI. Mental health professionals should not wait for chronic medical conditions to become acute and life-threatening to intervene; they should get involved way before and help people with SMI manage these conditions and even help prevent them in the first place. The clarification of professional boundaries and duties is also in line with current national and global efforts to increase the integration of health and mental health services for people with SMI and for developing medical homes for people with SMI within mental health settings because such facilities are usually their only source of medical care and their most frequented service sector (Alakeson et al., 2010).

Eliminating health care inequities among people with SMI is a tall order that will not be accomplished with one simple intervention, program, or

policy. As described in this chapter, these inequities arise from a multitude of interacting factors, from the way services are organized and configured to how people with SMI interact with and are treated in these systems of care. Solving these inequities requires attacking this problem from multiple angles, from different perspectives, with multiple approaches. What is needed are critical system-level transformations and reforms that build bridges over the chasm that separates the health and mental health care systems, bridges that integrate health care and mental health care, treating the whole person, focusing on both the mind and the body. Within our systems of care, we also need to improve the way health and mental health providers deliver health care to people with SMI to end stigma and discrimination, engender trust, and provide high-quality care for all. Moving beyond the clinic walls, we need interventions that help people with SMI engage in health-promoting behaviors in their everyday lives. As discussed in the next section of this book, there are numerous promising solutions for improving the health and health care of people with SMI. In the following chapters, I draw from the work my team and I have conducted adapting and testing different types of interventions (e.g., healthy lifestyle intervention, health care management) that aim to improve the physical health of people with SMI. I also discuss the work of other dedicated researchers and clinicians working in this field. By no means are these all the interventions being developed, tested, and deployed to reduce health inequities in people with SMI. It is beyond the scope of this book to describe all these interventions. Interested readers can refer to excellent systematic reviews for a more comprehensive description of this ever-growing literature (Cabassa et al., 2017; McGinty et al., 2015a; Siantz & Aranda, 2014). We will now move from problems to potential and promising solutions.

5

Engaging in Healthy Lifestyles

Sometimes the best interventions are not developed by scientists working in universities or medical centers using the most advanced technologies, therapeutic techniques, or the best controlled conditions. Sometimes the best interventions come from the field, from the desire to address growing health inequities and injustices, from the necessity to solve real-world problems in real time. People who are closer to the ground, who manage agencies or deliver care, often see, feel, worry about, and bear witness to the grim realities of going to too many memorial services and seeing their clients die young. It is out of these realties that some health interventions for people with serious mental illness (SMI) are created. The development of the In Shape program is one of these stories.

In Shape stands for Individualized Self-Health Action Plan for Empowerment (Van Citters et al., 2010). It is a health promotion program that aims to help people with SMI who are overweight or obese improve their health through exercise and healthy eating (Van Citters et al., 2010). As discussed in Chapter 2, poor dietary habits, lack of physical activity, high rates of obesity and smoking, and the weight gain and negative cardiometabolic side effects linked to the use of second-generation antipsychotics contribute to the poor health of people with SMI. In Shape aims to counteract these unhealthy behaviors. It was developed from a partnership between Kenneth Jue, the director, at that time, of a community mental health clinic in New Hampshire, and a research team from Dartmouth University led by Dr. Stephen Bartels. The program was first described in the *Community Mental Health Journal* (Van Citters et al., 2010). I first learned about In Shape through this publication and in a talk Dr. Bartels gave at the National Institute of Mental Health (NIMH) Mental Health Services Research Conference in Washington, DC. I also had the opportunity to interview Stephen about how this program took shape.

Stephen is a geriatric psychiatrist deeply interested in the intersection of physical and mental health. As he put it, "There is no mental health without physical health and no physical health without mental health; the two are

Addressing Health Inequities in People With Serious Mental Illness. Leopoldo J. Cabassa, Oxford University Press.
© Oxford University Press 2023. DOI: 10.1093/oso/9780190937300.003.0005

intimately intertwined." He has had an illustrious and productive career as a clinician, director of mental health programs, academic researcher, and mentor to many mental health researchers and scholars. He has worked in the public mental health system for decades. Stephen was the clinical director of a mental health center and was later appointed as the medical director of the mental health system in New Hampshire. It was through these positions and experiences that his commitment to address, as he calls it, "the greatest health disparities in the nation that people don't talk about, which is early mortality in people with mental illness," was crystalized. As he recounted during our telephone interview:

> One of my jobs was to review untimely deaths . . . reviewing too many mortalities in people in their 40s and mostly in their 50s. They weren't due to suicide and they weren't due to car accidents; they were due to heart disease. So . . . at that time, it harkened back to my fundamental interest in the interaction between physical and mental health, and I started getting very curious about what we could do in New Hampshire to address this.

It was during this period in Stephen's career that he connected with Kenneth Jue, who at that time was running the Monadnock Family Services in Keene, New Hampshire. Ken, much like Stephen, was deeply concerned about the physical health of his clients, about "going to too many funerals" as Stephen recalled. They connected at a meeting with the executive directors of mental health centers in New Hampshire. Ken approached Stephen and told him that he had started an interesting project called In Shape by putting together different elements to address his clients' health needs and hopefully help reduce the alarming premature mortalities he was seeing.

First, Ken had gone down the street from his clinic and begun a collaboration with Keene State College to get students from their physical education program to serve as health coaches to his clients. This partnership provided students real-world practical experience while at the same time helping Ken's clients. Ken then went to his local YMCA and got free gym memberships for his clients, which enabled Ken's clients to gain access to exercise equipment in their communities. Lastly, Ken began to connect his clients to smoking cessation programs to address the high rates of smoking at his clinic. By bringing these pieces together, Ken had developed the foundations of a health promotion program for people with SMI. His approach for developing this program came from the ground up. He identified a growing local need that required

immediate attention and then went about finding practical solutions by using existing community resources and assets.

As Stephen learned about this program, he wanted to study it to see if it worked.

I said [to Ken], "I'm a researcher, are you studying it?" He said, "Oh yes, we're doing satisfaction measures." I said, "No, are you studying it?" And it was at that point where I said, you know this is very important. This looks very interesting; giving people health coaches, giving people free gym memberships, having the coaches be trained both in physical fitness, but also in smoking cessation and particularly tailoring what we do for people with mental health challenges sounds like this has a future.

Stephen told Ken at that time, "I'll donate my time. We'll write grants ... and we will study this; because I think this is a very future focused program." This was the beginning of a long-standing partnership and decades of collaboration. What started as a community-based program turned into a manualized intervention that has been pilot tested (Van Citters et al., 2010) and became the basis for two randomized controlled trials (Bartels et al., 2013; Bartels et al., 2015), a statewide implementation project (Bartels et al., 2018), and a national implementation trial (Aschbrenner et al., 2019).

In Shape's main components include individualized weekly sessions with a health mentor who is a certified personal trainer, the use of fitness and diet plans tailored to the individual's needs, free access to local fitness facilities (e.g., YMCA), individual and group nutritional education, and referrals to smoking cessation programs. Health mentors help participants track their progress, set realistic goals, and stay motivated. In Shape's philosophy is grounded in the principles of recovery, self-determination, self-direction, inclusion, and health promotion (Van Citters et al., 2010). A key element of this program is that all activities occur in the community, which means that In Shape participants learn how to make healthier choices where they live and to use available resources to engage in a healthier lifestyle.

The evidence supporting In Shape's effectiveness in improving the physical health of people with SMI is strong. It is one of the few health interventions for people with SMI that has been rigorously tested, and its results replicated in multiple randomized clinical trials. The first trial was conducted in New Hampshire and enrolled 133 participants with SMI and a body mass index (BMI) greater than 25 (Bartels et al., 2013). Participants were randomized

to either In Shape or receiving a free 1-year fitness club membership. At 12 months, In Shape participants reported greater fitness club attendance, more participation in physical activity, statistically significant increases in vigorous physical activity, and greater improvements in dietary habits than participants in the comparison condition. Moreover, twice as many In Shape participants as those in the comparison condition (40% vs. 20%, respectively) achieved clinically significant improvements in cardiorespiratory fitness (CRF): "the ability of the circulatory and respiratory systems to supply oxygen to working muscles during sustained physical activity" (Vancampfort et al., 2015, p. 132). CRF is an important health indicator because it is strongly predictive of obesity, cardiovascular disease (CVD), and all-cause mortality in the general population and in people with SMI (Kodama et al., 2009; Vancampfort et al., 2015).

The second In Shape trial was conducted in Boston, enrolled a larger ($N = 210$) and more racially and ethnically diverse sample of people with SMI who were overweight or obese, and examined outcomes at 12 and 18 months after randomization (Bartels et al., 2015). It had a similar comparison condition as in the previous trial. The results from this second trial were more impressive. Compared to the comparison condition (free gym membership), In Shape participants reported greater weight loss and improvement in CRF at 12 and 18 months, suggesting that the impact of In Shape was sustained 6 months after the end of the 12-month program. Furthermore, at 12 months 51% of In Shape participants, compared to 38% in the comparison condition, achieved clinically significant reductions in cardiovascular risk by either reporting clinically significant improvements in CRF or clinically significant weight loss, defined as weight loss of 5% or more from the start of the trial. This advantage in CVD risk reduction among In Shape participants was sustained at 18 months.

The beauty of In Shape is that it provides people with SMI with practical tools, resources, and encouragement to make healthier choices in their everyday lives. This intervention motivates people with SMI to gradually and safely engage in physical activity and to improve their dietary habits by using the resources available to them in their communities. In Shape exemplifies how an intervention developed *in* the community *for* the community can produce significant health benefits. This work demonstrates how with the right support, motivation, and resources, people with SMI can engage in healthy behaviors to achieve a healthier lifestyle and improve their cardiovascular health.

Healthy lifestyle interventions like In Shape are a common approach to improving the health of people with SMI. These are structured interventions that use behavioral techniques—such as goal setting, self-monitoring, and problem solving—to help people increase their physical activity, manage their weight, eat a healthier and balanced diet, and engage in health promotion activities (Bartels & Desilets, 2012; Cabassa et al., 2010). In the general population, healthy lifestyle interventions are a cornerstone to combat obesity and lower the risk for type 2 diabetes and CVD (Ali et al., 2012). For example, the Diabetes Prevention Program (DPP), a landmark multicenter study of adults at risk for type 2 diabetes in the United States, found that compared to placebo, a structured healthy lifestyle intervention and the medication metformin significantly reduced the incidence of diabetes by 58% and 31%, respectively (Knowler et al., 2002). In fact, the lifestyle intervention was more effective than metformin. Both interventions were also found to be effective in men and women and in racial and ethnic minoritized groups, although Black women in the lifestyle intervention group had significantly lower weight loss compared to other racial/ethnic and gender groups (Knowler et al., 2002; West et al., 2008). Moreover, a 10-year follow-up study confirmed that lifestyle intervention and metformin continued to prevent and delay the onset of type 2 diabetes among DPP participants (Diabetes Prevention Program Research Group et al., 2009).

Multiple systematic literature reviews, some conducted by our group, have found that healthy lifestyle interventions can help people with SMI (Cabassa et al., 2010; McGinty et al., 2015a; Verhaeghe et al., 2011). A key finding from these reviews is that the most effective healthy lifestyle interventions for people with SMI tend to use intensive, manualized programs that combine coached and structured physical activity and supports for dietary changes using behavioral techniques, and last 9 months or more (Bartels & Desilets, 2012). The impact of these interventions varies, but when implemented correctly they can help people with SMI lose weight, increase their physical activity, and improve the quality of their lives (Verhaeghe et al., 2011).

In our work, we have consistently found that people with SMI, as in the general population, want help losing weight and would participate in healthy lifestyle programs if they are made accessible, attractive, and relevant to them. In the Photovoice project described at the beginning of this book, in which we explored the health needs of people with SMI living in supportive housing agencies in New York City, we discovered that many of our participants had strong preferences for bringing healthy lifestyle interventions into these

settings. For example, a Black participant in her mid-50s with bipolar disorder who had been struggling with weight gain for years mentioned in one of our group discussions, "If I can find a place, somebody to help me lose the weight that will be a good plus for me. . . . If [the supportive housing where she lived] could get somebody here to help other tenants, that would be good." Another participant, a Black male in his late 40s recovering from major depression and a substance use disorder, also captured this sentiment during one of the photo-elicitation interviews we conducted as part of this study. He said, "This weight wasn't put on in one day and you're not going to take it off in one day. You need help to chart a course . . . to set up means of doing it a step at a time" (as qtd. in Cabassa et al., 2013, p. 624).

Stephen, during his In Shape trials, also mentioned having a very similar experience:

We did not have problems recruiting people. These were the easiest studies I've ever done; both of those studies, [in terms of] recruiting people, because when we said . . . would you like to have either a free gym membership alone or a free gym membership with a health coach? . . . we had people lining up at the door wanting to be in this study. And that's because you know, people with mental health conditions they voted with their feet about wanting wellness. . . . A lot of people with mental health conditions want what everyone else wants. . . . They want to be well. They want to be fit, and they want to be not suffering from chronic health conditions.

What these experiences indicate is that healthy lifestyle programs address fundamental health needs in the lives of people with SMI. Losing weight, changing dietary habits, and increasing physical activity are extremely difficult things. Healthy lifestyle programs help chart a course and provide people with SMI with behavioral tools and motivation to support them in this long and often difficult journey.

An important element of this work is that these healthy lifestyle interventions need to be adapted to the unique needs and realities of people with SMI. Healthy lifestyle interventions developed and tested in the general population cannot just be applied to people with SMI. We are learning that for these interventions to be effective with people with SMI, they need to consider the lives of this population, their environments, and the impact that their mental illness and their psychiatric treatments have on their health behaviors. Two exemplars of adaptations to healthy lifestyle interventions

for people with SMI are the work by Dr. Gail Daumit and her team at Johns Hopkins University in their Achieving Healthy Lifestyles in Psychiatric Rehabilitation (ACHIEVE) trial (Daumit et al., 2013), and our own work developing and testing a peer-led healthy lifestyle intervention (Cabassa et al., 2015; O'Hara et al., 2017).

The ACHIEVE trial evaluated the effectiveness of an intensive 18-month tailored behavioral weight loss intervention for people with SMI (Daumit et al., 2013). The trial was conducted in 10 outpatient psychiatric rehabilitation centers in Maryland. Their healthy lifestyle intervention consisted of structured group exercise sessions conducted two to three times a week and weekly group and individual weight management sessions. The exercise sessions were designed for sedentary people with gradual increases in the intensity and duration of physical activity with the goal of motivating people to engage in moderate-intensity aerobic exercise. The weight management sessions focused on helping participants reduce their caloric intake by avoiding sugar and sweetened beverages and junk food, eating five daily servings of fruits and vegetables, and choosing small portions and healthy snacks. Because the rehabilitation programs that participated in this study provided clients breakfast and lunch, the intervention team also advised the kitchen staff at these centers to provide reduced-calorie food, thus facilitating the availability of healthy meals to all participants.

Several adaptations to the ACHIEVE intervention were conducted to address the unique needs of people with SMI. To inform these adaptations, Dr. Daumit assembled a multidisciplinary team of experts, including kinesiologists, psychiatrists, nutritionists, and psychologists. She also used findings from a small pilot study they conducted in preparation for their larger effective trial to identify areas for refinement and adaptations. For example, to counteract the common impairments in memory, motivation, and executive functioning related to SMI, intervention lessons and information were divided into small components with frequent repetition, and frequently recurring exercise and weight management sessions were done throughout the program. This helped increase participants' comprehension and self-efficacy (Daumit et al., 2013; Vazin et al., 2016). They also used simplified tracking tools to help participants monitor key health behaviors (e.g., eating fruits and vegetables) and to reinforce intervention goals. To motivate participation, session attendance was incentivized with a point system in which participants could trade points for small reward items. To reduce stigma toward physical activity and barriers for accessing

safe places to exercise, group sessions were delivered at the rehabilitation centers and facilitated by trained interventionists who created a supportive environment. Lastly, to reduce barriers to healthy foods, healthy breakfasts and lunches were made available at each psychiatric rehabilitation center participating in this study.

The ACHIEVE trial had impressive findings. At 18 months, ACHIEVE participants lost an average of 7 lb. compared to the control group, who on average lost 0.4 lb. (Daumit et al., 2013). Moreover, ACHIEVE was associated with clinically significant weight loss for 32.5% of participants at 12 months and 37.8% at 18 months (Daumit et al., 2013). A unique finding of this trial is that in contrast to lifestyle interventions in the general population, the weight loss of ACHIEVE participants did not peak early in the intervention. In most weight loss trials, people tend to lose weight in the first 3 to 6 months and then regain the weight as the intervention progresses. In the ACHIEVE study, the intervention group continued to lose weight throughout the trial, with the biggest weight loss, on average, occurring at 18 months. These findings suggest that the pattern of weight loss for people with SMI may be different as it may take longer for them to engage in health behavior changes and for those changes to result in weight loss outcomes.

Another example of how to adapt a healthy lifestyle intervention to the needs and realities of people with SMI is the work our team has done developing and testing a peer-led healthy lifestyle program in supportive housing agencies (O'Hara et al., 2017). In this project, we wanted to address barriers for increasing the reach, accessibility, feasibility, and relevance of healthy lifestyle interventions for people with SMI who are overweight or obese. Like many evidence-based interventions, healthy lifestyle interventions for people with SMI are not easily accessible in routine practice settings serving this population.

To address this important gap in care, we first wanted to expand the setting where these interventions are delivered. Most of the time, as we have seen in the studies discussed earlier in this chapter, healthy lifestyle interventions for people with SMI tend to be delivered in clinical settings, like community mental health centers, outpatient mental health clinics, and psychiatric rehabilitation programs. For this project, we wanted to bring healthy lifestyle interventions closer to people's doorsteps to make these interventions more accessible to people with SMI and reduce access barriers. With that goal in mind, we partnered with supportive housing agencies where many people with SMI reside (Cabassa et al., 2015). Supportive housing is an

important service setting for people with SMI because it provides affordable community-based housing alongside health, mental health, and social services (Nelson & Laurier, 2010). These agencies serve people with a range of psychiatric and health conditions, thus reaching a broad segment of people with SMI. Supportive housing agencies in the United States are also moving toward integrating health interventions into their operations to address the growing chronic medical conditions of their clients (Henwood et al., 2013; Henwood et al., 2011). In fact, several ongoing programmatic and financial supports available through the current health care reforms linked to the expansion of Medicaid benefits, the implementation of the Affordable Care Act, and national programs like the Substance Abuse and Mental Health Services Administration-Health Resources and Service Administration (SAMHSA-HRSA) Primary and Behavioral Health Care Integration are facilitating this expansion of services within supportive housing agencies and other behavioral health organizations throughout the United States (Henwood et al., 2011).

Second, we wanted to expand the people who could deliver these interventions to improve their reach and make them more economically feasible for community organizations. In most studies, as we have seen, healthy lifestyle interventions are often delivered by professionals such as registered nurses, dieticians, social workers, doctors, psychologists, and counselors. In this project, we wanted peer specialists to deliver our intervention. Peer specialists are people with lived experiences recovering from SMI who receive training to support others in their recovery. This segment of the mental health workforce is growing, with more than 30 states in the United States having some level of Medicaid reimbursement for these positions, and the number continues to grow with the expansion of Medicaid and the implementation of the Affordable Care Act in the United States (Chinman et al., 2014; Davidson et al., 2006; National Association of State Mental Health Program Directors, 2014). Peer specialists also bring credibility, trust, and hope to people with SMI (Bochicchio et al., 2019; Cook, 2011) As we have noted previously:

> Peer specialists can expose clients to positive and credible role models who can tap into their own experiences to provide instrumental, informational, and emotional support; help translate the health intervention into clients' daily activities on ecological and cultural terms; and become credible coaches. (Cabassa et al., 2015, p. 2)

Our peer-led healthy lifestyle intervention was adapted from the Group Lifestyle Balance (GLB) program, an established, manualized, group-based intervention that aims to improve healthy dietary habits and increase physical activity (Kramer et al., 2009). GLB is derived from the DPP and uses health education principles and core behavioral techniques, like self-monitoring, problem solving, managing unhealthy social cues, and stress management, to support healthy lifestyle changes (Knowler et al., 2002; Venditti & Kramer, 2012). Following the GLB structure, our peer-led program consists of weekly core sessions for 3 months, bimonthly transition sessions for 3 months, and monthly maintenance sessions for 6 months, for a total of 22 sessions over the course of a year. Each session lasts approximately 60 minutes and is delivered by a trained peer specialist to a group of three to six participants in their housing agency with the option of receiving individual make-up sessions if sessions are missed.

In a small pilot study we conducted at a supportive housing agency in New York City between August 2013 and March 2014, we cofacilitated our intervention with peer specialists to two different groups of participants to learn how to deliver the intervention and how to work with peer specialists in this capacity. It also provided us the opportunity to examine the intervention's initial acceptability and feasibility and identify key adaptations to improve the relevance of our intervention to people with SMI living in supportive housing. This pilot study enabled us to gain first-hand experiences with the intervention, to see what worked and what needed to be modified, and to get a sense of how people in supportive housing react to this structured program. Pilot studies are great for this initial exploratory work as they provide the flexibility to try out different things and collect multiple sources of information without the constraints of a more structured, randomized study. Throughout this study, Kathleen O'Hara, a doctoral student at Columbia University at that time, and I collected multiple sources of data, such as meeting notes, focus group transcripts, and field notes, to capture what we were learning and to use this information to make intervention adaptations. We described the details and findings of this pilot study in an article led by Kathleen (O'Hara et al., 2017). Here, I summarize the key intervention adaptations we learned from this pilot study that informed the development of our peer-led healthy lifestyle intervention.

The first set of adaptations focused on enhancing participants' commitment to and initial engagement in the intervention. We noticed that for some people attending group sessions could be an issue, and some people needed

extra assistance in getting the required medical clearances to safely participate in a weight loss program. To address these challenges, we started offering individual make-up sessions to those participants who missed group
sessions. This introduced flexibility and enabled participants to remain
connected to the intervention when other situations (e.g., hospitalizations,
other medical appointments, job responsibilities) prevented them from
attending group sessions.

Obtaining a medical clearance from a physician is a necessary require-
ment for most healthy lifestyle interventions to ensure that the physical activities used in these interventions are safe for participants given their complex
physical and mental health conditions. During this pilot study, we quickly
learned that many participants did not have a regular source of medical
care, or if they did, they did not visit their primary care doctors on a regular
basis. To overcome these barriers, we had our peer facilitators and research
assistants help coordinate these medical appointments, and in some cases
they accompanied the participants to their appointment to obtain medical
clearance.

The second set of adaptations focused on simplifying the self-monitoring
tools that are a key element of these interventions. Our intervention requires
that people record their daily food intake and physical activity and keep track
of their weight on a weekly basis. This record provided participants with
concrete evidence of how much they were eating, the types of foods they
consumed, and how much or how little physical activity they did on a regular
basis. The goal of self-monitoring was to increase participants' awareness of
how diet, physical activity, and weight are interconnected. It also enhanced
the participants' motivation to make health behavior changes and track their
progress over time.

During our pilot study, we noticed that self-monitoring tasks were hard
for most participants because many forgot or found it hard to adhere to these
tasks on a consistent basis. To address these issues, we developed a menu
of individualized self-monitoring tools that participants could choose from
to address their needs. These included simplified monitoring tools that
used pictures for participants with low literacy and a list of apps they could
use with their smartphones. We also provided participants blank pocket-
size notebooks to jot down information about what they ate in a free form.
Another option we developed was using a monitoring log with the www.
chooseMyPlate.gov graphic for each meal of the day, allowing participants to
record what they ate throughout the day using simple checkmarks.

The third set of adaptations centered around building healthy eating patterns to address the challenges participants faced in modifying entrenched unhealthy dietary habits and to reduce financial limitations in purchasing healthy food options on a limited monthly budget. To address dietary habits, we taught participants how to accurately measure portion size using their own hands or common household objects (e.g., deck of cards). These simple strategies enabled participants to gain a global understanding of how many calories they were consuming and how they may cut calories from their diets. Peer specialists, themselves from diverse cultural backgrounds, were also instrumental in sharing with participants how they made dietary changes in culturally congruent ways like cooking vegetables with southern recipes or substituting high-fat ingredients like lard with vegetable oil to prepare traditional dishes without sacrificing flavor. To address economic barriers, we provided resources (e.g., New York City Greenmarket handouts) to help participants use their Supplemental Nutrition Assistance Program (SNAP) benefits to purchase healthy foods, such as fresh fruits and vegetables, and connected them to food pantries to stretch their food budget and reduce food insecurity throughout the month.

The fourth set of adaptations focused on helping participants improve their physical activity. Given that many of our participants were sedentary and did not have an established exercise routine, we moved the content on walking and using pedometers to monitor and increase their daily steps from Session 10 to Session 4 to get the participants moving early in the intervention. We also encouraged peer facilitators to provide individualized support to participants around physical activity during weekly weigh-ins at the beginning of each session and during in-between-session check-ins. Doing so helped participants find ways to be more active and to adjust their physical activity to their own needs. For example, for participants with arthritis, we encouraged them to do safe stretching and to find low-impact exercises, such as swimming at a public pool or a local YMCA. We also developed apartment-based exercise options, such as dancing to music or walking in their apartments, to provide participants with ways to stay active during inclement weather or when they did not feel safe going outside to exercise. We provided participants a list of no- and low-cost resources, like gyms, public pools, and local parks and trails, to encourage them to engage in regular physical activity in their neighborhoods. Peer specialists offered their time to accompany participants on walks or to the gym to further encourage them to engage in physical activity. These strategies focused on addressing

common barriers people with SMI face when trying to engage in physical activity due to comorbid health conditions (e.g., arthritis), lethargy, and lack of motivation due to their mental illness and the side effects of psychiatric medications, inclement weather, lack of safe places to exercise, and lack of resources for exercising.

The last set of adaptations we learned from this pilot study revolved around making the behavioral strategies used in our intervention more salient and individualized for our participants. Behavioral strategies such as managing environmental and social cues, reducing self-defeating thoughts, developing relapse prevention plans, managing stress, and problem solving are core elements of our healthy lifestyle intervention. To increase the relevance of these strategies, we used individualized support in-between-session contacts and weekly weigh-ins to support participants in learning how to best match and use these behavioral techniques to address eating and exercise challenges. For instance, some participants liked to discuss their self-defeating thoughts with our group facilitators during our weekly weigh-in sessions, particularly when they failed to lose weight or had reached a weight plateau. This conversation created concrete spaces to address specific challenges in a personalized manner. We also encouraged participants to support and motivate each other given that support from others is an important approach for helping people during health behavior changes. Lastly, peer specialists used their in-between-session contacts either in person, via telephone, or by text to provide additional support and motivation to participants beyond the structured group sessions.

While we conducted this pilot study, we applied for a large grant from the NIMH to expand this work and support a larger and more rigorous evaluation of our intervention. Our proposal was eventually funded, and in July 2014 we embarked on a multiyear study to test the effectiveness and examine the implementation of our peer-led healthy lifestyle intervention in three supportive housing agencies. This was my first major National Institutes of Health grant, and it provided me the opportunity to partner with and hire Dr. Ana Stefancic as the project director. Ana has been an incredible partner in this journey. She is a clear-headed, steady, and determined leader; an excellent scientist; and a dedicated and passionate advocate for improving the lives of people with SMI. With her support and leadership, we assembled an incredible team of investigators, collaborators, students, research assistants, peer specialists, and community partners. This project has been an amazing journey, with many ups and downs along the way, but all in all we have

learned an enormous amount about the lives of people with SMI and how to work with peer specialists and supportive housing agencies to improve the health of this population. None of this work could have been accomplished without Ana's expertise, support, and leadership, and the dedication, passion, and hard work of our incredible team.

In July 2019, we completed this large pragmatic effectiveness trial of our peer-led group lifestyle balance (PGLB) intervention in three supportive housing agencies, two in Philadelphia and one in New York City. We enrolled 314 participants with SMI who were overweight or obese and randomly assigned them to either usual care (UC) or PGLB. Most of our sample (82%) were racial and ethnic minorities, mostly Blacks and Latino/as. Independent research assistants employed by the study team not blinded to the participants' group assignment conducted face-to-face interviews at the participants' supportive housing agency at baseline and 6, 12, and 18 months after randomization. Measurement protocols and instruments are described elsewhere in a protocol paper (Cabassa et al., 2015). We retained 80.3% (n = 252) of our original sample at 18 months. Our main hypothesis for this trial was that compared to participants receiving only UC, a significantly larger proportion of participants receiving PGLB would achieve clinically significant weight loss (e.g., at least a 5% weight loss from baseline), improvements in CRF (50-meter or more increase from baseline), and reductions in CVD risk at 12 and 18 months after randomization regardless of study site.

We found that after controlling for site and baseline weights, a higher proportion of PGLB participants compared to UC achieved clinically significant weight loss at 12 months (PGLB = 28.9% vs. UC = 24.3%) and 18 months (PGLB = 32% vs. UC = 30.8%), yet these differences were not statistically significant (Cabassa et al., 2021). Study outcomes differed by study site. At Sites 1 and 2, UC did better than PGLB at all time points on our main outcome, but these differences were not statistically significant. Site 3 showed a different pattern. At this site, PGLB was better than UC, including clinically significant reductions in CVD at 12 months (PGLB = 59.3% vs. UC = 32.7%, adjusted odds ratio [AOR] = 2.99, 95% CI [1.33, 6.72]) and clinically significant weight loss at 18 months (PGLB = 41.7% vs. UC = 21.7%, AOR = 2.57, 95% CI [1.02, 6.49]) (Cabassa et al., 2021).

The findings emerging from our trial suggest that PGLB benefits were not uniform across study sites. Differences across study sites are a common outcome in pragmatic trials, such as ours, given the clinical, organizational,

and community complexities of conducting these types of studies in routine practice settings (Davidoff, 2009; Dixon-Woods et al., 2011). In our trial, these complexities included conducting our study in three supportive housing agencies with different program philosophies (e.g., housing first vs. treatment first) and housing arrangements (e.g., scattered apartments vs. congregate housing), employing peer specialists rather than clinicians to deliver PGLB, and conducting the study in two cities (New York City and Philadelphia) with different health care systems and policies. Adding to these contextual complexities, we recruited a racially/ethnically diverse sample, mostly non-Hispanic Blacks and Latino/as, with complex physical, social, and mental health issues. For example, 91% were receiving SNAP benefits and were unemployed. On average, participants reported 3.6 chronic medical conditions (e.g., diabetes, hypertension) and were taking 1.7 psychiatric medications, mostly second-generation antipsychotics. Most of our participants had not only SMI but also a history of substance use disorder. These complexities provide a rich source of information to understand how and why our intervention worked in certain settings and not others, but more studies are needed to fully understand these complexities to inform future efforts to implement our intervention in other supportive housing agencies and behavioral health organizations in the community. Clarifying what worked for whom and under which conditions is critical because it can help future implementation efforts know what resources and actions are needed to successfully implement PGLB (Dixon-Woods et al., 2011). This is the next step in our line of research.

As we have seen, these healthy lifestyle interventions combine multiple components to support healthy behavior changes, such as helping people set and sustain realistic goals; teaching people how to regularly monitor their diets, weight, and physical activity; helping people build healthy dietary habits through portion control, calorie counting, and reducing fat and calorie intake; and eating more fruits and vegetables. They also teach people how to manage and successfully cope with difficult situations and combat self-defeating thoughts, teach how to use problem-solving techniques to address relapse, and provide social support and motivation to achieve and maintain weight loss and health goals (Venditti & Kramer, 2012). Currently, two questions that need to be addressed are which of these components do people with SMI find most helpful in supporting healthy lifestyle changes, and what aspects of these interventions do they value most? Answers to these questions are important as they can help identify the intervention elements

that are most effective, useful, and relevant for supporting the health of people with SMI.

Several interesting qualitative studies examining the experiences of people with SMI who have participated in healthy lifestyle interventions and successfully benefited from these programs are beginning to shed some light on these important questions (Aschbrenner et al., 2013; Shiner et al., 2008; Vazin et al., 2016). Qualitative methods, like in-depth one-on-one interviews and focus group discussions, are well suited to answers these questions because they provide participants an opportunity to tell their stories and describe in their own words what matters most to them. These methods capture the experiences of participants in these interventions, which can shed light into the aspects of these programs that they find most useful, relevant, and helpful as they engage and incorporate healthy lifestyle changes into their daily routines.

An interesting approach taken by some of these qualitative studies is that they focus on the participants who achieved some level of weight loss, thus learning from the people who benefited most from these interventions. For example, Shiner et al. (2008) from the Department of Psychiatry at Dartmouth Medical School interviewed participants from one of the early In Shape studies who had lost at least 10 lb. or had a reduction in waist circumference of at least 10 cm. Similarly, Roza Vazin and colleagues from the Bloomberg School of Public Health at Johns Hopkins University (2016) published a study in the *Psychiatric Rehabilitation Journal* in which they interviewed participants from the ACHIEVE trial who had lost weight during their participation in this intervention.

These and other qualitative studies (Aschbrenner et al., 2013; Hawes et al., 2022; Yarborough et al., 2016) provide several important insights into what people with SMI find most helpful and relevant from healthy lifestyle interventions. At a practical level, participants reported learning about concrete strategies they could use to change their diets and develop healthy eating patterns, such as reducing portion sizes in each meal, eating more fruits and vegetables, and drinking water instead of sugary drinks. Another key element was to gain free access to community gyms and exercise equipment and to have supportive staff who taught them how to exercise in a safe and supportive environment. Participants also appreciated how the physical activity elements of these interventions were tailored to their needs and how concepts and lessons were introduced gradually so that they could work out at their own pace and skill level.

Participants mentioned that the relationships they developed with the people who delivered these interventions were critical to their success. They talked about how facilitators provided them direction, structure, support, and encouragement in a nonstigmatizing manner that kept them engaged and motivated to make healthy lifestyle changes. Lastly, participants valued intervention benefits that went beyond losing weight and improving their health, such as improving their physical appearance, gaining self-confidence and a sense of accomplishment, and increasing their ability to perform activities of daily living. These benefits helped them with other aspects of their lives like forming new relationships, trying new things, and being more social and less isolated, thus contributing to their own recovery from mental illness, as captured by Mr. S's experience with our peer-led healthy lifestyle intervention.

Mr. S's story, summarized below, was chronicled in an online blog written by Will O'Brien (2016) from Project Home, a supportive housing agency in Philadelphia (for more details about the blog see https://projecthome.org/news/shawn-brown-healthy-balance). In 2015, Mr. S enrolled in our PGLB study (Cabassa et al., 2015). At the time of our study, he had SMI and diabetes and was obese. His weight was also exacerbating his inflamed knees and bad back. When describing how he felt at that time, Mr. S mentioned that he "often felt sluggish and down on himself."

Reflecting on his experience participating in PGLB, Mr. S mentioned, "It wasn't easy at first" to change his diet and engage in regular physical activity, but with determination and the support and encouragement from his peer specialist and the other participants in his group, he began to see his weight improve, and, as he put it, "something was working." Through the lessons learned in PGLB, Mr. S talked about how he began to slowly change his diet by eating more fruits and vegetables, practicing moderation and portion control, and reducing his consumption of fast foods. He described how PGLB enabled him to "have a better respect for food." Participating in PGLB also helped him become more physically active by exercising regularly and establishing an early-morning biking routine along a bike path near his home. Mr. S mentioned how biking was "exhilarating to be along the river early morning. I love it, it is my therapy."

Mr. S's engagement in the PGLB program resulted in substantial weight loss and better control of his diabetes. It also benefited Mr. S in other aspects of his life beyond his health, including his ongoing recovery from SMI and improving his relationships with family and friends. For Mr. S, PGLB was

not a temporary program; it represented an important turning point for breaking his cycles of unhealthy behaviors and embracing a healthier balanced lifestyle as captured by this sentiment when describing how PGLB had changed his outlook: "I am not getting any younger, and I want to be around a lot longer. I want to keep this balance. I want to be a person who is easy to get along with."

Mr. S's story and the evidence of the positive impact that healthy lifestyle interventions can have on the health of people with SMI are a testament of what is possible with the appropriate supports, resources, and determination. It shows that the cycles of unhealthy behaviors in unhealthy environments that negatively impact the health of people with SMI can be broken and that healthy habits can be established. Mr. S's story can inspire other people with SMI and chronic medical conditions to change their lifestyle. In his own words, "If I can be an influence for someone, I will definitely show them what kind of results are possible." Increasing the life expectancy of all people with SMI requires that we continue to bridge the gap between research and practice and develop the evidence on how to best implement healthy lifestyle interventions in routine practice settings to increase their accessibility, reach, and benefits.

6
From Fragmentation to Integrated Care

Health care managers can save lives. In the summer of 2015, during a routine visit to her health care manager, Marta arrived complaining of shortness of breath and chest pain. Marta at that time was in her mid-50s and had multiple medical conditions including high blood pressure, high cholesterol, and prediabetes along with schizoaffective disorder. She was a participant in a study we were conducting at an outpatient mental health clinic in New York city (Cabassa et al., 2016). Marta was born in Puerto Rico but had lived in the mainland United States for most of her life. She did not finish high school and lived alone in a small apartment in upper Manhattan. Marta never married and had two daughters who lived nearby. Marta spoke mostly Spanish but could understand some English.

Several weeks before her visit, Marta had undergone a minimally invasive surgical procedure. The procedure reduced Marta's pain. After surgery, she was feeling well and resumed her day-to-day actives. In fact, before this visit she was looking forward to attending her younger daughter's birthday.

Up to this point, Marta had participated in our study for about 6 months and had developed a trusting relationship with Felipe, her health care manager. In this project, we were examining whether master's-level social workers could deliver a year-long health care manager intervention that our team had adapted from an existing health care manager program to address the health care needs of people like Marta, who were mostly Spanish-speaking Latino/as with serious mental illness (SMI) and at risk for cardiovascular disease (CVD). In this intervention, which we called *Puentes Para Mejorar Su Salud y Bienestar* (Bridges to Better Health and Wellness), health care managers do not provide direct medical services; instead, they work individually with patients in their mental health clinic to engage and connect them with primary care services. The goals of our program were to increase patients' receipt of preventive primary care, such as receiving screenings and vaccinations, to improve their quality of life and hopefully reduce their risk for CVD. Health care managers motivate and encourage patients to engage in their own medical care and serve as coordinators and facilitators between

Addressing Health Inequities in People With Serious Mental Illness. Leopoldo J. Cabassa, Oxford University Press.
© Oxford University Press 2023. DOI: 10.1093/oso/9780190937300.003.0006

patients' primary care and mental health providers. Health care managers are the bridge to ensure no one falls through the cracks as patients navigate between these two systems of care.

During this latest visit, Felipe noted that Marta was tearful and looked sluggish as she explained her symptoms. Marta disclosed experiencing pain radiating from her ear to her chest for the past 3 to 4 days and said "*respiro come si me falta aire*" (I breathe but I'm lacking air). Two things alarmed Felipe. First, Marta rarely complained of pain, and she looked tired and drained, which was unusual because she was always full of energy. Second, chest pain and shortness of breath are two symptoms that, based on our program's protocol, required Felipe to consult a medical provider at the clinic, usually a nurse or the participant's psychiatrist, for immediate medical evaluation. These two symptoms are usually indicators of more serious health problems.

Felipe alerted Marta's psychiatrist, who evaluated her and determined she needed to go to the nearest emergency room (ER). Working with Felipe, Marta's psychiatrist wrote a brief letter alerting the ER doctor of Marta's medical history, recent procedure, and current symptoms and medications. Felipe then proceeded to find Marta transportation to the ER. Because Marta refused to go on an ambulance, Felipe paid for a taxi and called one of Marta's daughters to meet Marta at the ER. He stressed to Marta's daughter the urgency of the situation and developed a follow-up plan whereby Felipe would call Marta's daughter to get an update on the situation and to make sure Marta was getting the care that she needed. A few minutes after establishing this plan and with a letter in hand, Marta was escorted into a taxi and traveled to the nearest ER.

After several hours, Marta's daughter called Felipe from the hospital reporting that Marta was admitted to the intensive care unit (ICU) because her evaluation revealed that she had three pulmonary emboli. Marta's daughter also told Felipe that the ICU doctors had expressed how Marta was very fortunate to receive immediate care because due to the severity of her symptoms, it was unlikely that Marta would have survived much longer without an emergency intervention. Her daughter was thankful for Felipe's quick action and support because Marta had been reluctant to seek medical attention as she did not want to burden her daughters with her medical problems and did not want to miss her younger daughter's birthday. Marta spent the next 2 weeks in the hospital recovering from this incident. Marta's story is an example of how a routine visit to a health care manager can save a life.

Health care manager interventions are one of the many approaches used to help people with SMI get medical care when they need it. These interventions aim to reduce the fragmentation of care that people with SMI often experience as they navigate between the mental health and health care systems. Health care managers' responsibilities are multifaceted and are designed to reduce the numerous barriers that people with SMI face as they seek, engage, and use medical care. They prevent people with SMI from falling through the enormous cracks that exist in our health care system by increasing the access and use of high-quality medical care.

In their most basic form, health care managers serve as a bridge between patients and their primary care and mental health providers, creating partnerships with all of them to ensure patients' health issues are being properly identified, evaluated, treated, monitored, and managed. For patients, health care managers serve as coaches and advocates. They partner with patients to teach and model the skills necessary for problem solving and goal setting. Coaching patients is an ongoing process that focuses on solidifying and strengthening patients' self-management skills so that they can implement them independently and at the right times to get the care they need. Health care managers work with patients, and whenever possible their family members, to develop and carry out an activation plan, including identification of objectives to achieve their overall health goals and identification of potential barriers. As health care advocates, health care managers work closely with patients to help mobilize the necessary resources and supports so that patients receive the health care that they need.

For mental health and primary care providers, health care managers serve as a bridge, facilitator, and coordinator of care. Health care managers work closely with patients to assess and monitor their medical needs as they relate to specific health issues, such as preventive primary care and cardiovascular health, and share this information with providers. As facilitators, health care managers follow screening and monitoring guidelines for preventive primary care and common cardiometabolic indicators (e.g., blood pressure, weight, blood glucose levels) and alert mental health and primary providers of abnormal values and health issues that arise, as well as track and monitor patients' progress. As coordinators, health care managers work closely with providers to connect patients to medical care and report back to providers for follow-up care.

Health care manager interventions make intuitive sense and have strong appeal because they use a dedicated professional, usually a registered nurse

or social worker, to help remove the many obstacles that prevent people with SMI from accessing high-quality medical care. The evidence supporting the use of health care managers to improve access and receipt of high-quality care is strong and growing. One of the best studies rigorously testing the impact of health care manager interventions in a community mental health clinic serving people with SMI is the Primary Care, Access, Referral and Evaluation (PCARE) project conducted by Benjamin Druss and colleagues (2010) from the Rollins School of Public Health at Emory University. In fact, the health care manager intervention that helped Marta, Bridges to Better Health and Wellness, was informed by PCARE and is an adaptation of the health care manager intervention that Dr. Druss and his team developed and tested in his trial.

In PCARE, 407 adults with SMI receiving mental health care at a community mental health clinic in Atlanta, Georgia, were randomized to receive the usual care (UC) they received at this clinic for their medical needs or to receive a health care manager intervention. Most of the participants in this randomized controlled trial were Black (77%) and resided in economically disadvantaged neighborhoods with a median annual income of $3,400. The most common psychiatric diagnoses were schizophrenia, depression, and bipolar disorder, and one in four participants reported a co-occurring substance use disorder. The most common medical conditions that participants had when they enrolled in this trial included hypertension, arthritis, tooth or gum disease, and asthma.

The health care intervention used in PCARE included two full-time registered nurses working at the community mental health clinic. They followed a manualized health care manager protocol focusing on overcoming patients' barriers by providing them with information about their medical conditions, connecting them to primary care providers, and helping coordinate medical appointments. Health care managers were trained to use motivational interviewing skills to help activate and motivate patients to engage in their own medical care. They also used action plans, a common behavioral tool for helping patients identify needs and teaching them behavioral skills to enhance self-management strategies for achieving goals for medical care and/or healthy lifestyle changes (Handley et al., 2006). For providers, health care managers helped advocate for patients' care, shared information with providers, and developed care coordination plans. They also coached patients to prepare them to have better interactions with their medical providers. In some instances, health care managers accompanied patients to their medical

visits. The health care managers met monthly with patients, and the intervention lasted 12 months. In contrast, UC at this mental health clinic consisted of providing participants with a list of available primary care providers in the community that accepted Medicaid insurance.

The key outcome in this trial was the receipt of preventive primary care services using 25 indicators derived from the U.S. Preventive Services Taskforce Guidelines, including physical examinations (e.g., eye exams, blood pressure), screenings (e.g., cholesterol, HIV), vaccination (e.g., influenza), and education services (e.g., smoking cessation). Other outcomes examined included receipts of care for common cardiometabolic conditions (e.g., diabetes, hypertension); presence of a primary care provider other than relying on ER care; and health-related quality of life. Outcomes were measured at baseline and 12 months after randomization.

In an article published in the *American Journal of Psychiatry*, Druss and colleagues (2010) reported that at 12 months participants who were randomized to receive the health care manager intervention doubled their receipt of preventive primary care from 21.4% at baseline to 58.7%, while the preventive primary care received by participants randomized to receive UC remained basically the same during this time period (21.6% to 21.8%). In fact, compared to UC, there were significant increases for participants receiving the health care manager intervention in all the preventive primary care indicators examined in this study. For example, from baseline to 12 months, screenings (e.g., cholesterol, HIV) increased from 22.4% to 50.4%, physical examinations (e.g., blood pressure, eye exams) increased from 32.9% to 70.5%, and vaccinations increased from 3.1% to 24.7%. Moreover, the health care manager intervention showed that they successfully connected people to primary care and increased their visits to general medical providers. This increase resulted in a significant increase in the identification of previously undiagnosed medical conditions, particularly hyperlipidemia and hypertension. Among participants with one or more cardiometabolic conditions (e.g., diabetes), the health care manager intervention increased the receipt of indicated services for these conditions from 26.6% at baseline to 34.9% at 12 months, whereas those in the UC condition basically stayed the same at 27.7% through this entire period. Lastly, participating in the health care manager intervention compared to UC increased participants' mental-health-related quality of life. The findings of the PCARE study are impressive and provide compelling evidence that a manualized health care manager intervention employing registered nurses at a community mental health clinic

can produce meaningful improvements in the quality of medical care for people with SMI.

In our work, we built upon PCARE results and adapted their health care manager intervention for people such as Marta, Latino/as with SMI and at risk for CVD, using master's-level social workers instead of registered nurses to increase the fit of this much-needed intervention in our local community. Social workers are a natural fit for taking on the role of health care managers in community mental health clinics because they deliver most of the mental health care in the United States (Ivey et al., 1998), many can bill for care manager functions in mental health treatment settings, and social workers have an established history of working closely with historically marginalized racial and ethnic minority communities. Social workers also bring expertise in counseling, care coordination, and system navigation, matching the required skills for effective health care management (Cabassa et al., 2011).

Our adaptation of the PCARE intervention was informed by working closely with a community advisory board composed of social workers, a primary care physician, a psychiatrist/clinic administrator, and a peer specialist and by findings from a mixed-methods study in which we use a combination of structured interviews, focus groups, and chart abstractions to examine the views of Latino/a patients with SMI about their primary care experience (Cabassa, Gomes, Meyreles, Capitelli, Younge, Dragatsi, Alvarez, Nicasio et al., 2014). Results of this study generated several critical findings that informed the adaptations we made to the health care manager intervention used in PCARE to address the unique needs of Latino/as with SMI. First, we found that compared to previous studies, our Latino/a clients reported that the quality of care they received from their primary care doctors was poor. They also reported lacking confidence in how they could manage their own chronic illnesses, such as diabetes and hypertension, and did not feel that they were active participants in their own care. These findings suggest that Hispanics with SMI are prime candidates for health care manager interventions that target care coordination, goal setting, patient activation, and self-management.

Second, we captured how participants experienced high levels of perceived discrimination and stigma from primary care providers due to their ethnicity, immigration status, SMI, and the intersection of these historically marginalized identities in the U.S. health care system (Cabassa, Gomes, Meyreles, Capitelli, Younge, Dragatsi, Alvarez, Nicasio et al., 2014). These findings point to the need to create better bridges between primary

and mental health care to help reduce providers' stigma and biases. They also highlight the importance of having health care managers serve as advocates for Latino/a patients to ensure they get the medical care they need when they need it. Finally, participants' relationships with their primary care providers revealed that Hispanic clients preferred clinicians who displayed an interpersonal style compatible with the core cultural norms valued by many Latin American and Caribbean cultures, such as *personalismo* (being warm and personable and showing that personal ties outweigh formal, institutional connections), *respeto* (respect), and *dignidad* (dignity) (Cabassa, Gomes, Meyreles, Capitelli, Younge, Dragatsi, Alvarez, Nicasio et al., 2014). These interpersonal styles informed how we trained our health care managers to relate and present themselves to Latino/a patients and how to best interact with these patients. Embedding these cultural norms into the training and supervision practices we used with the health care managers in our study served as the foundation that our health care managers used to establish and eventually solidify trusting relationships with their Latino/a patients.

We then put the adapted intervention to a small feasibility test. We conducted a 12-month pilot study with a sample of 34 Latino/as with SMI and at risk for CVD using a single group pre–post design to test the acceptability, feasibility, and initial impact of our culturally adapted health care manager intervention, Bridges to Better Health and Wellness, in a public outpatient mental health clinic using social workers (Cabassa et al., 2016). We wanted to know whether these clients found the intervention useful and relevant, whether master's-level social workers could successfully deliver the intervention, and whether participating in this intervention resulted in better health care outcomes.

Eighty-five percent of the people who initially enrolled in our study completed the 12-month intervention, and on average, participants attended 10 of 12 monthly sessions with their health care manager. We found that our culturally adapted intervention was associated with statistically significant improvements of moderate to large effect sizes on patient activation, self-efficacy, and patients' assessments of chronic illness care, and significantly increased the receipt of preventive primary care services (e.g., vaccinations, screenings) over a 12-month period, from 29.9% at baseline to 54.9% at 12 months (Cabassa et al., 2016).

To gain a deeper understanding of participants' experiences with Bridges to Better Health and Wellness, we also conducted three focus groups with participants who completed the intervention (Cabassa et al.,

2019). Results from these group discussions indicated that what mattered most to participants was the health education they received, the positive relationships they formed with their health care managers, the care coordination assistance they obtained, and the motivation and activation they gained from this intervention. Participants consistently expressed forming deep personal connections with their health care mangers, as captured by Marcela, a participant of Dominican descent with diabetes and bipolar disorder, who described her relationship with her health care manager in the following way: "She treated me very well, like I was family. . . . She talked to me with such humility, she was very open, and I thank God that I had her for a year. . . . She was always so open with me, always with a smile on her face, always very professional" (Cabassa et al., 2019, p. 1229). What we learned from participants' own words was that key elements of Bridges to Better Health and Wellness, such as care coordination and the motivation, encouragement, and assistance participants got from their health care managers, were central to shaping their experiences with this intervention and beneficial for addressing their health care needs.

Despite the positive results of health care manager interventions in improving the receipt of preventive primary care and in linking people with SMI to medical care in times of need, these interventions tend to have limited impact in improving objective health outcomes. For example, the PCARE study showed no differences between the health care manger intervention and UC in improving blood pressure and reducing cholesterol levels, two important and objective indicators of cardiovascular health (Druss et al., 2010). We also had a similar result in our Bridge to Better Health and Wellness study. Participants at the end of a year working with our health care managers did not report any improvements in weight or blood pressure.

What we are learning from studies examining the impact of health care manager interventions is that to improve objective health outcomes in people with SMI and reduce the risk for CVD, more intensive interventions may be needed. It may not be sufficient to just connect people to medical care; we need to improve the actual care that people receive to improve the health outcomes directly linked to premature mortality in people with SMI.

A potential solution to this gap in health care is the development of behavioral health homes for people with SMI. This model of delivering and organizing physical health care services for people with SMI and chronic medical conditions aims to integrate and embed different types of health services (e.g., screenings, care coordination, care management)

in specialty mental health organizations, such as outpatient mental health clinics or community mental health centers (Fortuna et al., 2020). The goal of behavioral health homes is to place the responsibility for coordinating, managing, and in some cases delivering most of the physical health care of people with SMI on specialty mental health organizations rather than on the primary care clinic (Murphy et al., 2018). The specialty mental health sector, as we have seen throughout this book, is a critical venue for people with SMI because it is usually the main point of care for this population, and the providers in this sector have expertise working with people with SMI and tend to form long-standing relationships with these clients (Alakeson et al., 2010). As described in previous chapters, people with SMI often face stigma and discrimination in primary care settings due to the lack of experience primary care providers have working with this population and in addressing and managing their complex health and mental health needs.

Behavioral health homes are not a standardized intervention. In fact, this complex integrated model of care can take on many forms, and the level of service integration can also vary (Murphy et al., 2018). For example, some behavioral health homes employ and embed a health care provider, such as a nurse practitioner, in the specialty mental health clinic. Others use health care managers, usually registered nurses or social workers, to help with screenings, referrals, and care coordination. Others combine these approaches and provide nonclinical services such as self-management classes, smoking cessation groups, or behavioral weight loss programs. Despite these different configurations, the unifying features of behavioral health homes are that they tend to place a strong emphasis on screening, care coordination, tracking and monitoring patients' progress, using a multidisciplinary team to address patients' health care needs, and using a patient-centered, whole-person approach to improve the health and general well-being of people with SMI (Alakeson et al., 2010). The foundations that support behavioral health homes are built upon the chronic care model, which focuses on redesigning how health care is configured and delivered to address chronic illnesses, such as diabetes and hypertension. The chronic care model aims to provide patients with ongoing health education and self-management supports for their conditions. It also empowers providers with decision supports and accessible clinical information systems to track patients' progress, conditions, medications, treatments, and interactions with multiple providers. It links patients to community resources, such as housing assistance, social services,

and other community-based agencies needed to support their well-being (Stanhope & Ashenberg Straussner, 2018).

Behavioral health homes have proliferated throughout the United States due to multiple federal and state initiatives. As discussed in Chapter 2, in 2009 the Substance Abuse and Mental Health Services Administration launched the Primary and Behavioral Health Care Integration program, a large-scale national initiative supporting the implementation of behavioral health homes (Scharf et al., 2013). Moreover, as of this writing 17 states and the District of Columbia have implemented behavioral health homes with support from the Affordable Care Act Medicaid Health Home Waiver and the Center for Medicare and Medicaid Innovation demonstration projects (Daumit et al., 2020). The most common behavioral health home configurations under these programs tend to be located in community out-patient mental health centers that include formal organizational and financial partnerships with federally qualified health care centers that provide primary care services to poor and historically marginalized communities (Druss et al., 2017).

Given that behavioral health homes have become a leading approach for improving the health care of people with SMI in the United States, what do we know about their effectiveness? Do they help people with SMI receive preventive primary care services? Do they improve the quality of medical care in this population? Do they reduce the risk for CVD and improve important objective health indicators linked to premature mortality in people with SMI? A recent article by Dr. Karen Fortuna and colleagues (2020) from Dartmouth provides some important answers to these questions.

In this article, the team conducted a systematic literature review of peer-reviewed studies examining the impact of behavioral health homes on service utilization (e.g., use of primary care services, use of ERs), receipt of preventative screenings (e.g., blood pressure, laboratory tests for fasting blood glucose and cholesterol levels), and impact on cardiometabolic risk factors measured via objective measures (e.g., blood pressure, blood glucose, body mass index [BMI]). All studies included in their review compared the behavioral health home to another group, which included other health home models, UC services, or matched samples. The review included 18 articles—11 observational studies, four quasi-experimental trials, and three randomized controlled trials.

Most of the reviewed studies showed that behavioral health homes tend to increase screening for preventive services (e.g., diabetes screening,

mammograms, HIV screening) and help people with SMI connect to routine medical care. Fortuna et al. (2020) also found that behavioral health homes reduced the use of ER visits, particularly in studies conducted outside the Veterans Administration system. However, the effectiveness of behavioral health homes on improving health outcomes seems to be mixed and inconclusive at this time, with some studies showing improvements in certain cardiometabolic risk factors (e.g., systolic blood pressure, weight) but not in others (e.g., total cholesterol, HbA1c; Druss et al., 2017; Putz et al., 2015).

Based on Fortuna et al.'s (2020) review of the existing literature, they concluded that behavioral health homes can help improve access and quality of health care for people with SMI. Yet these improvements are not enough to significantly improve health outcomes and reduce early mortality in people with SMI. Like health care manager interventions, more needs to be done to address the complex health inequities faced by people with SMI. Fortuna and colleagues recommended a series of enhancements to behavioral health home models that could help combat these health inequities. First, the focus of behavioral health homes should be on screening and intervening. Behavioral health homes need to clearly standardize and implement treatment guidelines that help providers identify health problems, especially those that focus on cardiometabolic conditions, and provide evidence-based clinical guidance on how to proactively treat and manage these conditions. Second, the interventions and clinical services included in behavioral health homes need to not just target improvements in cardiometabolic indicators, such as helping people lose weight or reduce their blood pressure, but focus on achieving clinically significant thresholds for the myriad conditions linked to CVD. For example, providers in behavioral health homes should use a treat-to-target approach for achieving blood pressure control among people with hypertension or help stabilize glucose levels for people with diabetes. Treat to target is a common strategy for treating multiple chronic medical conditions that combines the careful monitoring of patients' laboratory values on key health indicators (e.g., blood pressure, cholesterol or glucose levels) to determine the adjustment of pharmacological and/or behavioral treatments following treatment guidelines until a predetermined target in these laboratory values is achieved (Chwastiak et al., 2014). This strategy will enable behavioral health homes to personalize the care that they deliver to the specific health needs of the people they serve. Third, more attention needs to be paid to using interventions, approaches, and services that target multiple interdependent risk factors (e.g., obesity, smoking, diabetes) at once given

the interconnection of risk factors and health conditions linked to the poor health of people with SMI. The impetus here is to provide a comprehensive package of interventions that aims to improve cardiovascular health from multiple angles. Lastly, Fortuna et al. found that behavioral health homes that included elements of peer support and training in self-management skills showed the greatest reductions in cardiometabolic risk factors. They recommend that these elements be included as core components of behavioral health homes. These recommendations are all sensible, but the question remains whether they will achieve the goal of improving the physical health of people with SMI.

Findings from a recent randomized clinical trial led by Daumit and colleagues (2020) from Johns Hopkins University provide some initial answers to this important question. In this study, they tested whether a comprehensive 18-month intensive intervention that combined behavioral counseling for cardiovascular health, care coordination, and care management could significantly reduce the risk of CVD in adults with SMI who also had at least one cardiovascular risk factor, including hypertension, diabetes, dyslipidemia, current tobacco smoking, and/or being overweight or obese, compared to only receiving UC.

They recruited 269 people with SMI drawn from four outpatient psychiatric rehabilitation programs in Maryland. Their intervention used self-management concepts and social cognitive theory to promote health behavior change around the American Heart Association's Life Simple 7 for improving cardiovascular health that focuses on managing blood pressure, controlling cholesterol levels, reducing blood sugar levels, increasing physical activity, eating better, losing weight, and stopping smoking. Health coaches and nurses worked individually with participants to reduce their overall risk of CVD. The intervention also included care coordination and care management in which nurses shared critical health information with participants' medical providers, facilitated the scheduling of appointments, and in some instances accompanied patients to their doctor's appointments. The health coaches and nurses met individually with participants and used patient-centered approaches to facilitate behavioral change. They also used a point system to reward participants for attendance and to incentivize healthy behavior changes, like smoking cessation.

The primary outcome of this trial was change in the risk of a cardiovascular event using the global Framingham Risk Score from baseline to 18 months.

The Framingham Risk Score estimates the 10-year probability of a cardiovascular event (e.g., coronary heart disease, cerebrovascular event, heart failure) by examining a series of modifiable risk factors associated with CVD (e.g., smoking, total cholesterol, systolic blood pressure) and personal characteristics (e.g., age, gender) linked to heart health (Daumit et al., 2020). Compared to participants receiving only UC, which entailed connecting people to primary care services, the intervention group reported a 12.7% relative risk reduction in the 10-year probability of a cardiovascular event. In other words, people who received the comprehensive intervention significantly reduced their chances of having a cardiovascular event, like a heart attack or stroke, in the next 10 years compared to those who just received UC services at these programs. A driving factor for this important finding was that a larger proportion of people in the intervention group quit smoking throughout the trial compared to those in the UC group. Moreover, improvements in blood pressure and cholesterol levels also contributed to the overall risk reduction in cardiovascular events in the intervention group compared to the UC group.

The results of this trial provide important evidence that combining behavioral counseling that targets multiple CVD risk factors all at once using the American Heart Association's Life Simple 7, care coordination, and care management can produce clinically significant reductions in the risk for CVD in people with SMI. Incorporating and implementing this type of comprehensive program into behavioral health homes could be an effective approach for improving the health and health care of people with SMI.

As discussed in this chapter, improving the health of people with SMI requires that our health care system end the delivery of fragmented care; provide people with SMI the tools, resources, supports, and opportunities they need to manage their complex physical health conditions; and implement integrated models of health care. Like Marta, all people with SMI should have access to a health care manager who can help them connect with the appropriate medical care in times of need. However, integrating health and mental health care may not be enough to improve the health of people with SMI. As captured by Druss et al. (2017), "Better quality [health care] alone may be insufficient to improve more distal medical outcomes" (p. 8). To reduce the deadly and unnecessary health inequities that disproportionately impact people with SMI, the latest evidence points toward implementing a

multifactorial package of health services that empowers people with SMI with the skills and resources to proactively manage their chronic health conditions and reduce behavioral risk factors, improves care coordination, facilitates system navigation, and provides care management throughout the entire continuum of care.

7

Smoking

The Elephant in the Room

Smoking is the elephant in the room as it is a major contributor to premature mortality in people with serious mental illness (SMI), but compared to other health issues it has received limited attention. For years, our team shared this same blind spot as we focused most of our work on other health needs of people with SMI, such as increasing physical activity, losing weight, and improving the access, quality, and coordination of medical care. However, looking back at our different projects, smoking cast a long shadow on the lives of our participants. For example, in our Bridges to Better Health and Wellness health care manager study described in Chapter 6, about a third of participants reported being current smokers (Cabassa et al., 2016). More recently in our peer-led healthy lifestyle study in supportive housing agencies, described in Chapter 5, about 60% of participants were smokers (Cabassa et al., 2020). In the original proposal for this book, I did not include a chapter on smoking or smoking cessation because I have not done work in these areas. But as I began writing this book and delved deeper into the health inequities of people with SMI, I came to realize that I could no longer ignore one of the deadliest risk factors impacting this population. This chapter focuses on discussing the elephant in the room and grabbing it by the tail to improve the health of people with SMI.

The evidence that smoking is a major contributor to the poor health and early mortality of people with SMI is overwhelming. Compared to the general population, smoking rates are 2 to 5 times higher in people with schizophrenia, bipolar disorder, major depression, and posttraumatic stress disorder (Prochaska et al., 2017). It is estimated that people with mental illness consume nearly half of all cigarettes sold in the United States, with similar consumption patterns reported in the United Kingdom, Australia, and New Zealand (Prochaska et al., 2017). To compound the matter, SMI is associated with heavy smoking (e.g., consuming 25 cigarettes or more per day), elevated prevalence of nicotine dependence, and lower quit rates (Prochaska

Addressing Health Inequities in People With Serious Mental Illness. Leopoldo J. Cabassa, Oxford University Press.
© Oxford University Press 2023. DOI: 10.1093/oso/9780190937300.003.0007

et al., 2017; Stubbs et al., 2015). People with SMI who smoke also report lower quality of life, poorer mental health, worse cognitive functioning, and worse functional outcomes compared to nonsmokers with SMI (Depp et al., 2015; Dickerson et al., 2013). People with SMI tend to start smoking at an earlier age than the general population. For example, in some studies more than half (58%) of people with first-episode psychosis tend to be smokers, a significantly higher prevalence than people of similar age without psychosis (Firth et al., 2019). Because tobacco smoking disproportionately impacts people with SMI, leaders in the field consider smoking as one of the most significant yet challenging modifiable risk factors negatively impacting the health of this population, requiring urgent attention (Stubbs et al., 2015).

Smoking is arguably the number one killer of people with SMI because it is linked to the leading causes of early mortality and poor health (e.g., cardiovascular disease, cancer) in this population. Of the approximately 520,000 annual tobacco-related deaths in the United States, it is estimated that more than 200,000 are among people with mental illness, with most being people with SMI (Prochaska et al., 2017). The evidence is even grimmer regarding the causes of death of people hospitalized for severe psychiatric disorders. For example, in a large study of over half a million people hospitalized for a mental illness in California between 1990 and 2005, Russel Callaghan and colleagues (2014) discovered that about half of the total deaths of people hospitalized for schizophrenia, bipolar disorder, or major depression during this time period were due to diseases linked to tobacco use (e.g., cancer, cardiovascular disease, respiratory diseases). Sadly, this deadly health inequity continues to grow in people with SMI as the prevalence of smoking among people with schizophrenia and bipolar disorder continues to increase, while the prevalence of smoking in the general population continues to decline (Dickerson et al., 2018).

The reasons for this alarming inequity in smoking in people with SMI are multifactorial, complex, and not completely understood. Three general hypotheses have been stipulated (self-medication, causal effect, and shared vulnerability), yet the evidence is not conclusive and cannot fully explain the relationship between smoking and SMI (Sharma et al., 2016). The self-medication hypothesis stipulates that people with SMI smoke to relieve their symptoms and reduce side effects of antipsychotic medications, such as cognitive impairment and Parkinsonian symptoms. However, the evidence indicates that smoking often begins before the onset of schizophrenia and does not have antipsychotic properties; in fact, smoking may increase some

symptoms (e.g., depression, anxiety, hallucinations) and has been associated with greater illness severity and lower quality of life among people receiving treatment for first-episode psychosis (Oluwoye et al., 2019; Prochaska et al., 2017; Sharma et al., 2016). Smoking can also stimulate the metabolism of some psychiatric medications, thus leading to lower therapeutic blood levels and increasing the need for higher dosages (Prochaska et al., 2017). The causal hypothesis stipulates that smoking may cause SMI because it often precedes the onset of psychiatric conditions. However, few rigorous prospective studies have tested this hypothesis, and the link between smoking and SMI may be confounded by the association between smoking and use of other substances (e.g., cannabis) linked to the onset of psychosis (Sharma et al., 2016). Lastly, the shared vulnerability hypothesis stipulates that smoking and SMI may have common genetic and environmental causes; however, existing studies only point toward potential common factors and do not provide strong evidence for these shared causal pathways (Sharma et al., 2016).

Despite this inconclusive evidence, these hypotheses point toward certain factors that can help inform smoking cessation interventions and policies for people with SMI. One critical area is the negative and dismissive attitudes and beliefs that many mental health clinicians have toward smoking and about the ability and motivation of people with SMI to quit or reduce their smoking. For example, in a meta-analysis of 38 studies that included 16,396 mental health providers, Kate Sheals and colleagues (2016) from University College in London found that 42% of providers included in these studies reported serious barriers to smoking cessation interventions, such as lacking basic knowledge and training about smoking cessation and expressing low confidence in their ability to help their patients quit smoking. Forty percent reported negative attitudes toward smoking cessation, including that quitting smoking could have a negative impact on patients' symptoms or recovery, that patients may not be interested in quitting smoking, and that smoking cessation treatment was not part of their professional roles. More alarming was that almost half (45%) of mental health professionals in these studies reported endorsing tolerant attitudes toward smoking, such as endorsing the belief that smoking is an important coping mechanism for people with mental illness, that smoking helps patients establish a therapeutic relationship, and that quitting smoking is too much for patients to handle, among others. The tobacco industry propagated and endorsed some of these beliefs by actively disseminating marketing materials and funding research pushing

the self-medication hypothesis and falsely claiming that smoking reduces psychiatric symptoms (Prochaska et al., 2017). These efforts fueled higher smoking rates in people with mental illness (Prochaska et al., 2017). Overall, the findings from Dr. Sheal et al.'s meta-analysis indicated that many mental health clinicians may not feel comfortable discussing smoking cessation with their patients and their misapprehensions may deter them from offering advice, support, encouragement, and referrals to smoking cessation treatments.

A study led by researchers from the Department of Psychiatry at Washington University School of Medicine in St. Louis, highlights how discrepancies in attitudes toward smoking between patients with SMI and their providers negatively impact the receipt of smoking cessation treatments. In this study, Li-Shiun Chen and colleagues (2017) examined the interest of patients in receiving and mental health providers in offering smoking cessation treatments in four outpatient community mental health clinics in Missouri. The results of this exploratory study were published in the *Community Mental Health Journal*. Dr. Chen and her team at Washington University in St. Louis found that almost half of patients with SMI who currently smoked expressed being interested in receiving smoking cessation treatments, yet only a third received these treatments. Patients and their mental health providers also had different views about smoking cessation. Despite the fact that the majority of people who smoked (82%) in this study reported interest in quitting or reducing their smoking, the majority of psychiatrists (91%) and case workers (84%) reported that low patient interest was a major barrier for offering smoking cessation interventions to their patients. Other common barriers reported by mental health providers in this study included doubts that patients would comply with treatments, lack of training and referral sources (even though U.S. Food and Drug Administration [FDA]-approved smoking cessation medications such as nicotine replacement therapy [NRT], varenicline, and bupropion were available at the community mental health clinic pharmacies at no cost to patients if prescribed by their psychiatrists), and lack of time. These findings illustrate the different views that people with SMI who smoke and their mental health providers hold about quitting smoking and how these discrepant attitudes may prevent some providers from offering the supports and treatments people with SMI need and want to help them reduce and ultimately quit smoking. In fact, studies have shown that people with mental disorders are as motivated to quit smoking as the general population (Siru et al., 2009).

Despite these differences in attitudes, a systematic literature review and meta-analysis published in *General Hospital Psychiatry* found that people with and without mental illness tend to receive comparable rates of smoking cessation advice from their providers (Mitchell et al., 2015). In fact, rates of smoking cessation advice were similar for people with schizophrenia and bipolar disorder compared to people in the general population without these mental disorders. These findings highlight a troublesome trend in which the smoking cessation advice people with SMI receive from their medical providers is not proportionate to their needs. People with SMI should be receiving higher rates of smoking cessation advice from their providers than the general population given the high prevalence rates and harm from smoking in this population (Mitchell et al., 2015).

More proactive efforts are needed to educate all mental health providers on smoking cessation treatments and provide them with the necessary tools and skills to help them engage and motivate their clients to quit smoking (Stubbs et al., 2015). Since 2008, the Public Health Service Guidelines and the American Psychiatric Association have encouraged psychiatrists and other mental health professionals to receive training in the treatments for tobacco use (American Psychiatric Association, 2006). In fact, treatment guidelines recommend that all clinicians use the "5 A's" (ask, advise, assess, assist, and arrange) to engage patients who smoke in smoking cessation treatments (Chen et al., 2017). The impetus of these efforts comes from studies showing that brief advice from health care providers to quit smoking is associated with a significant increase in the likelihood that smokers will engage in smoking cessation (Prochaska et al., 2017). Given that outpatient mental health settings are at the heart of care for people with SMI and are the setting they tend to visit the most, each visit with a mental health provider—be it with a psychiatrist, social worker, psychologist, peer specialist, or care manager—is a critical opportunity to reinforce the health benefits of reducing and quitting smoking (Chen et al., 2017; Prochaska et al., 2017).

Yet the uptake of these guidelines and the training of mental health professionals on smoking cessation have been slow. In a national study that surveyed representatives from 114 psychiatric residency training programs from 40 U.S. states, Washington, DC, and Puerto Rico, Judith Prochaska and colleagues (2006) from Stanford University found that approximately half of participants reported that they had a tobacco cessation curriculum with a median duration of 1 hour. About 43% offered their residents clinical experiences for treating nicotine dependence in people with mental illness,

and most of the content (95%) of these training programs focused on pharmacological treatments (Prochaska et al., 2006). To address this major gap in training, the School of Pharmacy, University of California at San Francisco (2022) developed Rx for Change, a free web-based training curriculum for tobacco cessation grounded on the principles set forth by the U.S. Public Health Service Clinical Practice Guideline for Treating Tobacco Use and Dependence. The goal of this program is to equip health professionals with evidence-based knowledge and skills for assisting smokers with SMI to quit smoking in a safe and supported manner. This type of free training should be mandatory for all mental health clinicians.

Given the elevated rates of smoking in people with SMI, what do we currently know about smoking cessation approaches for this population? A variety of smoking cessation interventions are available to help people with SMI quit smoking. Multiple systematic literature reviews and meta-analyses indicate that there are at least three main pharmacological approaches recommended for people with SMI: NRT, bupropion, and varenicline (Peckham et al., 2017; Stubbs et al., 2015). NRT commonly comes in a range of forms—as a patch, gum, inhaler, or nasal spray—and provides low levels of nicotine concentration that help reduce withdrawal symptoms linked to physical dependence. Bupropion (brand names Wellbutrin, Zyban, and others) is an antidepressant that has nicotine-receptor-blocking activity. Varenicline (brand names Chantix and Champix) is a partial agonist of the α4β2 neuronal nicotinic acetylcholine receptor, which inhibits the binding of nicotine, thus reducing withdrawal symptoms while at the same time decreasing the pleasurable or reinforcing effects of smoking and other tobacco products.

Existing clinical guidelines also indicate that combining these cessation medications with behavioral counseling is safe, is well tolerated, and can optimize and support quit rates in smokers with SMI (Evins et al., 2015). Different behavioral approaches that can be delivered in individual or group settings or through technology-based platforms (e.g., websites, smartphone applications, telephone quit lines) include cognitive behavioral therapy, motivational interviewing, supportive counseling, and contingency management (e.g., provision of cash incentives to encourage and sustain abstinence; Brunette et al., 2020). Evidence to date indicates that the combination of pharmacological treatments and behavioral interventions is the most promising approach for helping people with SMI quit smoking without worsening their psychiatric symptoms (Brunette et al., 2020; Evins

et al., 2015). However, the evidence is inconclusive at this time in identifying which combination of pharmacological and behavioral treatments is the most effective in helping people with SMI quit smoking and sustain their abstinence. In fact, people with SMI need guidance from their clinicians in determining which smoking cessation treatment will be the best for them given their unique needs, psychiatric treatments, potential negative interactions with psychiatric medications, and personal preferences (Ferron, Brunette, He, et al., 2011).

In an article published in *Lancet Psychiatry*, Simon Gilbody and colleagues (2019) from the Department of Health Sciences at the University of York presented the results of a large randomized pragmatic trial conducted in the United Kingdom that highlighted the state of the evidence in smoking cessation treatments for people with SMI. In this trial, they tested the effectiveness of a smoking cessation intervention adapted for people with SMI, called SCIMITAR+, versus usual care (UC). They recruited 526 adults with bipolar disorder or schizophrenia who smoked at least five cigarettes a day from 16 primary care and 21 community-based sites in the United Kingdom. The adapted intervention provided participants with behavioral support from a mental health smoking cessation practitioner and pharmacological treatment (e.g., NRT, varenicline). Key adaptations for people with SMI included making several assessments before setting a quit date, offering NRT before setting a quit date, recognizing the purpose of smoking in the context of a person with SMI, providing home visits and face-to-face support after unsuccessful quit attempts or relapses, and informing the participants' primary care doctor and psychiatrist of a successful quit attempt so they can review and adjust antipsychotic medications doses. UC consisted of accessing the free smoking cessation services provided by the participants' primary care doctors or mental health clinicians, including pharmacological treatment available at these clinics, and accessing the free telephone helpline (Smokefree National Helpline). None of these UC services were adapted for people with SMI.

The primary outcome for this study was the percentage of people who stopped smoking at 12 months using a standardized objective indicator that combined self-report cessation for the previous 7 days and a carbon monoxide measurement below 10 parts per million. Dr. Gilbody and colleagues found that the proportion of people who quit at 12 months was slightly higher in the intervention group compared to those only receiving UC (15% vs. 10%, respectively), but the difference between the two groups did not

reach statistical significance. However, significant improvements in quit rates and health-related quality of life were reported for the intervention group compared to the UC group at 6 months. Another important finding from this study was that there was no significant deterioration of mental health symptoms between the two study conditions, providing further support that offering smoking cessation is not detrimental to the mental health of people with SMI. In all, Gilbody et al.'s study demonstrated that with appropriate supports, people with SMI can and do engage in smoking cessation and that adapted smoking cessation treatments can significantly increase quit rates in the short term (by 6 months) in this population. Yet, similar to the general population, it is hard to demonstrate long-term smoking cessation results, and thus more supports and efforts are needed to capitalize on these important findings.

Expanding the reach, use, and uptake of existing smoking cessation approaches is the next frontier for helping more people with SMI quit smoking. Dr. Mary Brunette's work in this area represents, in my opinion, a great exemplar of the type of efforts, innovation, and passion needed to tackle this important public health issue. I had a chance to interview Mary over the telephone about her work and what inspired her to dedicate her career to improving smoking cessation treatments for people with SMI. Dr. Brunette is a psychiatrist specializing in addiction in people with SMI. One of the many unique attributes of Mary's work is that she is both an academic conducting rigorous mental health services research as an associate professor of psychiatry at the Dartmouth Geisel School of Medicine and an administrator in the public mental health system serving as the medical director of the Bureau for Mental Health Services for the New Hampshire Department of Health and Humans Services.

Her dedication to helping people with SMI quit smoking crystallized early in her career. As she discussed during our telephone conversation, it was around 2006 when she began her position as medical director. One of her tasks as director, as she described it, was to "review all the reports of people who had died [within the public mental health system in New Hampshire], including their whole story, their reasons for death, and what had happened." The goals for conducting these reviews were to look for patterns and problems in their system of care so that they could from an administrative perspective "make changes that would reduce the likelihood that this would happen again." During one of these reviews Mary came across one of her previous patients. "I picked up my stack of papers for that day and whose

name did I see . . . [a patient] who I had worked with for 5 years," as she mentioned during our interview. "He had died at a young age of a heart attack. He was [someone] I had worked closely with for quite some time, who I was very fond of, and I was sad that he had died." Mary talked about how she had helped this patient recover from his mental illness and addiction, but he also smoked. In reviewing this case, she reflected on how she had offered him help with quitting smoking, as she did with all her patients, but stated, "I never pushed it as much as I felt I should have; I felt like, you know, I could have done more."

This case helped Mary place a human face to the grim statistics she was reviewing as the medical director and to the emerging studies and reports she was reading in the literature at that time describing the elevated rates of premature mortality in people with SMI. As she described during our interview:

> But then as that year went on, it wasn't just [this patient]. Name after name
> came across my desk of people that I had worked with, helped them, who
> were dying young, not of suicide, but of chronic health conditions. They
> were all smokers and I felt like, you know what? I could have done more. If
> we had helped these people quit smoking earlier in their lives, they would
> not be dead right now. . . . So, I really dug into this idea of trying to more
> systematically and more robustly address smoking for people with serious
> risks. . . . That's why I started working with collaborators on this idea of de-
> veloping digital tools through which we could reach more people.

The idea for increasing the reach of smoking cessation treatments in people with SMI was also propelled by the findings from a study that Mary was involved in at that time with her colleagues from Dartmouth. In this study, Dr. Joelle Ferron and a team from Dartmouth (Ferron, Brunette, McHugo, et al., 2011) used longitudinal data from an existing project of 174 people with co-occurring substance use and SMI to explore their patterns of cigarette use and cessation attempts over 11 years. They found that at the start of their study, 89% of participants were current smokers, and most (75%) reported they had attempted to quit smoking at least once throughout this 11-year period. Despite these high rates of smoking and quit attempts, none of these participants received NRT or bupropion, and only a few (17%) reported not smoking at the 11-year follow up. This study clearly described the extent to which people with SMI in New Hampshire receiving mental health services lacked basic access to smoking cessation treatments.

What Mary learned from these findings, from her own work in the public mental health system in New Hampshire, and from what she was reading in the literature was that people with SMI, as she put it, "actually did want to quit" and that many attempted to quit on their own without accessing or being offered smoking cessation treatments. She concluded that her mental health system needed more systematic ways to "get people linked with treatment" and that a variety of technology-based tools could help bridge this gap in smoking cessation care for smokers with SMI.

The idea to use technology was also fueled by her own disillusionment with trying to address this problem by doing in-person training with clinicians. During our interview, Mary talked about how "training will not cut it"—there is too much staff turnover in the mental health system to be able to train everyone on smoking cessation practice. "We were worn out with training people. It just felt like it was endless and that we would never get there," she told me. Mary felt they needed a more efficient and effective approach. At that time, technology tools (e.g., websites) were advancing, and she felt they could be harnessed to "create durable strategies to either train clinicians or to directly deliver interventions to the consumer; [both] would be as effective and have a much greater reach . . . in a cost-effective way" than continuing to do in-person training with clinicians.

This desire led Mary to conduct a series of innovative projects developing and testing web-based technology tools that could be deployed in public mental health settings to help and motivate people with SMI engage in smoking cessation treatments. A good exemplar of her work in this area is the development and testing of Let's Talk About Smoking, a web-based intervention tailored for smokers with SMI that focuses on increasing their motivation to quit smoking using a series of evidence-based interactive approaches and techniques. Let's Talk About Smoking was carefully developed through an iterative process that included extensive input from people with SMI (Ferron, Brunette, McHugo, et al., 2011). This innovative web-based intervention starts by asking users to choose a male or female video host, who presents themselves as an ex-smoker with SMI. The host then guides the user through a series of interactive modules using personalized assessments and feedback, motivational interviewing techniques and exercises, and health decision tools designed to motivate the user to initiate smoking cessation treatments (Brunette et al., 2020). A cool feature of Let's Talk is the series of quit story videos of people using different cessation treatments. At the end of

the intervention, the user gets a personalized report highlighting their desire to quit, their treatment choices, and referral information.

In an article published in the *Journal of Medical Internet Research Mental Health*, Dr. Brunette and colleagues (2020) presented the results of the first randomized controlled trial comparing the efficacy of Let's Talk versus a static web-based smoking cessation patient education pamphlet developed by the National Cancer Institute (NCI). In this study, 162 current smokers with SMI 18 years of age or older were recruited from community mental health clinics in New Jersey, Massachusetts, and Illinois. Participants were randomly assigned to Let's Talk or the NCI patient education website and followed for up to 6 months. The primary outcome of interest of this trial was participants' use of a smoking cessation treatment verified via a review of clinic medical records.

Study results indicated that both interventions seemed to have worked as no significant differences between the two interventions were reported in getting participants to initiate smoking cessation treatments. About 38% of participants enrolled in this study used a smoking cessation treatment during the 6-month follow-up period. These rates of treatment initiation are consistent with the ones achieved by interventions using in-person approaches such as motivational interviewing (Brunette et al., 2020). Despite these null findings, participants rated the Let's Talk interactive intervention as more appealing than the NCI intervention. Overall, the findings from this initial randomized controlled trial suggest that web-based interventions seem to be feasible and acceptable and can produce comparable results in motivating people with SMI to initiate smoking cessation treatments as in-person interventions. More studies are needed to replicate these findings in a larger and more diverse sample of smokers with SMI and to better understand the impact and use of technology-based interventions for people with SMI.

Efforts to reduce smoking among people with SMI require innovative, creative, and feasible approaches that take into consideration the unique needs of this underserved population. Dr. Brunette's work adds to the growing efforts needed to eliminate this deadly risk factor in people with SMI. Her research and clinical work have demonstrated that technology-based tobacco treatments tailored for people with SMI are a tool to expand access and reduce barriers to these treatments, particularly in public mental health clinics that face multiple demands and workforce shortages. As she described during our interview, "There's no reason why we shouldn't be harnessing these tools to get effective interventions into the hands and minds of our consumers."

She is currently actively working with local providers and clinics in her mental health system to integrate these technology tools into their everyday work and to get these interventions used by clinicians and their patients in routine practice.

We can no longer ignore the public health imperative of helping people with SMI quit smoking. We need to attack this deadly risk factor from multiple fronts (Das & Prochaska, 2017). Combating smoking should be a central aspect of mental health care from the very beginning of treatment. At an early stage, we need to prevent people with SMI from becoming dependent on tobacco products. For people with SMI who smoke, cessation treatments need to be made readably available, free of cost, and easy to access. All mental health facilities need to be tobacco free, and training of all mental health clinicians from all disciplines in smoking cessation approaches and treatments should be the norm, not the exception. Given the burden, costs, and suffering caused by smoking in people with SMI, smoking cessation should be an essential treatment incentivized and covered by all insurance programs. To improve the health and increase the life expectancy of people with SMI, reducing the rates of smoking needs to be a priority.

8

Flattening the Mortality Curve

A Call to Action

> Addressing the poor clinical health and early mortality in [people with serious mental illness] will require multimodal strategies addressing the full range of risk factors that underlie these problems.
>
> —Druss et al. (2017, p. 8)

The original goal for this final chapter was to present a vision for the future full of lofty ideas, recommendations, and prescriptions for improving the health and life expectancy of people with serious mental illness (SMI). The plan was to bring together the lessons we learned from the people represented throughout this book, people like Carla, Miguel, Rosa, Enrique, Cristina, Isabel, Angela, Gonzalo, Mr. S., Marta, and Marcela; to draw general conclusions from the different health interventions and programs described in previous chapters; and to summarize the recommendations laid out in multiple reports and literature reviews focusing on how to best reduce premature mortality in people with SMI. But in the time of COVID-19 and the uprising for racial and social justice ignited by decades of structural racism and injustices and the murders of George Floyd, Breonna Taylor, and countless others (*que en paz descancen*) at the hands of police officers in the United States, these plans had to change. Instead of describing a vision, what is needed, in my opinion, is a call to action for fundamental and pragmatic changes to flatten the mortality curve in people with SMI and end these deadly health inequities.

But 2020 was a year like no other. It pulled back the curtains and clearly revealed the deep social, economic, political, and health inequities that have taken root in our society and how they directly impact our everyday lives. Since the beginning of 2020, a novel coronavirus spread to every corner of the globe. As of March 2022, more than 460 million people have been

Addressing Health Inequities in People With Serious Mental Illness. Leopoldo J. Cabassa, Oxford University Press.
© Oxford University Press 2023. DOI: 10.1093/oso/9780190937300.003.0008

infected, and more than 6 million people have died worldwide. In the United States, COVID-19 has infected approximately 79 million people and killed more than 960,000 people. Yet, infections and deaths continue to rise in the United States and around the globe.

This pandemic has disrupted everyone's lives, but like other infectious diseases COVID-19's burden, suffering, and deaths are disproportionately impacting historically marginalized communities in the United States For example, data from the U.S. Centers for Disease Control and Prevention (CDC) indicated that as of June 2020, 21.8% of COVID-19 cases were among Blacks and 33.8% were among Latino/as despite the fact that these groups make up 13% and 18% of the U.S. population, respectively (Tai et al., 2020). COVID-19 mortality rates are also elevated in racial and ethnic groups compared to non-Hispanic Whites. In Chicago, for instance, the mortality rate as of May 2020 was 73 per 100,000 in Blacks, 39 per 100,000 in Latino/as, and 22 per 100,000 in non-Hispanic Whites (Hooper et al., 2020). In New York City, age-adjusted COVID-19 death rates per 100,000 were almost double in Latino/as (236) and Blacks (220) compared to non-Hispanic Whites (110; Tai et al., 2020). In Arizona, Native Americans compose 5.3% of the state's population yet they account for 13% of COVID-19 cases and 18% of COVID-19-related deaths (Tai et al., 2020).

A more troublesome trend is emerging from the examination of excess deaths associated with COVID-19 in 2020. Excess deaths are an important public health metric as they capture the number of persons who have died from all causes beyond the expected number of deaths for a given time and place (Rossen et al., 2020). It is a measure that can help clarify whether more people are dying than what would be expected in a particular time period, such as 2020, compared to other years in a given place, in this case, the United States. Excess deaths are commonly used to ascertain the overall mortality impact of a public health crisis, particularly when it is not clear if the deaths that are being reported are directly caused by COVID-19 given existing limitations in diagnostic testing and potentially inaccurate reporting of causes of death in death certificates (Rossen et al., 2020).

Findings reported in the *Morbidity and Mortality Weekly Report* published by the CDC on October 15, 2020, estimated that 299,028 more people have died than expected between January and October 2020 in the United States, and about two thirds of these excess deaths were attributed to COVID-19 (Rossen et al., 2020). Even though every segment of our society experienced increases in mortality rates in 2020, the distribution of these excess deaths

shows deep racial and ethnic inequities (Figure 8.1). Compared to the average number of deaths reported between 2015 and 2019, the largest average percentage increase in excess deaths in 2020 has been among Latino/as with an average increase of 53.6%, followed by Blacks with an average increase of 32.9%, American Indians/Alaska Natives with an average increase of 28.9%, and non-Hispanic Whites with an average increase of 11.9%.

COVID-19 clearly exposed the long-standing health inequities that continue to plague historically marginalized communities in the United States. Given the growing health inequities in people with SMI discussed throughout this book, we can surmise that COVID-19 has the potential to exacerbate the poor health and premature mortality in this at-risk population. Most of the health risk factors that increase COVID-19 mortality, including diabetes, obesity, chronic obstructive pulmonary disease, and cardiovascular disease, and the social conditions associated with COVID-19 infections, morbidity, and mortality, like poverty, homelessness, and lack of access to medical care, are overwhelmingly present in people with SMI (Bartels et al., 2020). Add to these risks the fact that many people with SMI reside in places like congregate housing, homeless shelters, long-term care facilities, nursing homes, and psychiatric hospitals that elevate the risk for exposure and transmission of COVID-19, and you have on top of an already public health crisis a new

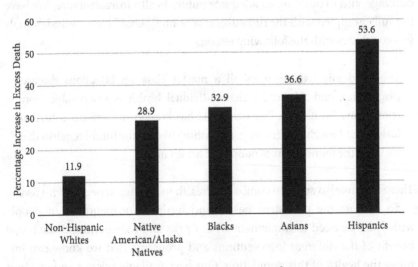

Figure 8.1 Percentage increase in excess death by race and ethnicity in the United States in 2020 compared to 2015–2019.

Note: Figure was orignially developed for this book presenting results reported in Rossen et al. (2020).

deadly hurricane brewing (Bartels et al., 2020). The urgency to combat health inequities in people with SMI can no longer be ignored or disputed. The time to act is now.

In the time of COVID-19, flattening the infection and mortality curves became a national imperative. Yet, as described by Dr. Atul Gawande (2020) in the *New Yorker*, the failure of the United States to truly flatten these curves can be characterized as "an implementation problem." Despite the fact that during most of 2020 there was no vaccine for this virus or well-established treatments for COVID-19, the country did have effective public health measures such as social distancing, testing, contact tracing, and wearing masks that could have controlled the spread of this virus and reduced infections, minimized deaths, and prevented suffering. In the United States, we were not able to successfully implement these public health strategies on a national scale. In his insightful analysis for why the United States was so slow and in-effective in developing a national approach to flatten the COVID-19 curves, particularly around testing and contact tracing, Dr. Gawande argued that it is "not simply that our national leadership is unfit [which it was under the Trump administration], but also that our health care system is dysfunctional." He further explained, "We are now paying the price of our long, uniquely American resistance to making sure that everyone has proper health-care coverage, and to building an adequate public-health infrastructure. We have not fully grappled with the difficulties we're up against." Dr. Gawande's analysis concludes with the following lessons:

> The pandemic has given us all a master class on infectious disease, diagnostics, and the reality that individual health is inseparable from community health. . . . The pandemic has brought Americans a further lesson: our best chance for long, flourishing lives in the future requires that we build the foundations of our public health now.

These lessons also apply to combating health inequities in people with SMI.

To address the persistent health and health care inequities in people with SMI, we need to implement what works and to expand the reach and benefit of the different interventions and programs that we know can im-prove the health of this population. Our best available science and our best clinical practices need to come together to help bridge the gaps that cur-rently exist in the access, quality, and outcomes of medical care for people with SMI. Fundamental and pragmatic reforms need to be implemented to

flatten the premature mortality curve that has caused so much unnecessary and preventable suffering and deaths in people with SMI. The suggestions and strategies that I describe in this chapter are by no means exhaustive, but I think they can make substantial progress in addressing these health inequities. These ideas build upon the existing recommendations that have been put forward in recent years by several research groups and government reports to improve the health of people with SMI (Firth et al., 2019; Liu et al., 2017; World Health Organization, 2018). This call to action is informed by our work with the people represented throughout this book and the lessons we learned from their stories and lived experiences with SMI and chronic medical illnesses. The ideas stipulated in this chapter are also shaped by what we have learned from the existing literature, and from the recommendations expressed by the dedicated colleagues, researchers, clinicians, and advocates we have met over the years working to improve the lives of people with SMI.

Health Prevention and Promotion From the Very Beginning

One of the clearest reforms needed to fundamentally shift the risk of poor health and premature mortality in people with SMI is to focus on physical health from the moment people are diagnosed with a mental illness and re- ceive their first psychiatric medication. In fact, when asked about what is the next generation of work that is needed to improve the health of people with SMI, almost everyone interviewed for this book agreed upon health pre- vention and promotion as major points. Stephen Bartels commented that there is a critical imperative to get ahead of these health inequities and get "people engaged early in the process" to focus on their health before these health problems take root. Gail Daumit observed that we "absolutely need prevention . . . where health is built into the system of care" from the start "so that people won't have these issues in the first place." Mary Brunette also expressed the critical need for getting "people to quit [smoking] young" and that the field should be focusing on prevention, not just mitigation. Moreover, as discussed by Kelly Aschbrenner, a fellow social worker, col- league, and associate professor of psychiatry at the Geisel School of Medicine at Dartmouth College who is conducting innovative health interventions for young adults with SMI using technology-based approaches (Aschbrenner et al., 2022), "We definitely need to work on even earlier intervention and

prevention" with adolescents and young adults and find the best ways to integrate "healthy [lifestyle] interventions as part of [early intervention] models."

The evidence is clear that the first years of treatment for a serious mental disorder like psychosis is a "critical period" for emerging cardiometabolic risk with significant increases in weight and worsening trends for blood pressure, glucose, cholesterol, triglycerides, and other cardiometabolic indicators (Correll et al., 2014; Pérez-Iglesias et al., 2014; Phutane et al., 2011; Srihari et al., 2013). It is also evident that helping people with SMI quit smoking early in their lives can have a profound positive impact in their health trajectory and reduce premature mortality, since quitting before people reach their 30s can reduce the deadly health consequences to levels similar to those of people who have never smoked (Gates et al., 2015). Furthermore, given all that is currently known about the weight gain and cardiometabolic side effects of antipsychotic and other psychiatric medications commonly used to treat SMI, there is no excuse for not proactively addressing physical health when delivering mental health care.

A prescription for an antipsychotic medication should be directly linked with a behavioral prescription that focuses on health prevention and promotion and equipping people with the health education and awareness coupled with the behavioral skills needed to make healthy dietary changes, increase physical activity, quit smoking if they smoke, and provide direct and easy access to preventive primary care. Physical health needs to be at the center of mental health care—they need to go hand in hand, not one without the other. As described in Chapter 3, people should not be forced to choose between their mental health at the expense of their physical health ("No Mental Health Without Physical Health," 2011). As mental health clinicians, we can no longer treat the negative health consequences of mental health treatments as just a series of side effects that needs to be screened and monitored and is someone else's responsibility to manage and treat. As exemplified in Jackie Curtis's program Keeping the Body in Mind for people with first-episode psychosis, the focus on health for mental health clinicians is to "not just screen but intervene" (Curtis et al., 2016).

Integrated Models of Care for People With SMI Should Be the Norm, Not the Exception

Another critical area for reducing the premature morality curve is to accelerate and ensure the implementation and sustainment of integrated models

of care like the ones described in Chapter 6. These models are designed to end the fragmentation and gaps in medical care that contribute to the excess morbidity and mortality in people with SMI by improving access to health screenings, preventive primary care, care coordination, and health care management resources. These models also deploy multidisciplinary teams and patient-centered approaches to help people with SMI successfully manage their complex physical health conditions. As we saw with Miguel in Chapter 1 and Marta in Chapter 6, integrated models of care can save lives by providing people with SMI with the appropriate supports and encouragements and by facilitating system navigation and connections to appropriate medical treatments in times of need. The implementation of integration models of care in routine practice settings for all should be a national priority.

We need to continue to harmonize the delivery of health and mental health care for people with SMI by making sure everyone has timely access to high-quality health care. As stipulated by the fundamental causes of disease theory, inequities in health are driven by the differential access to resources, such as knowledge, money, power, and beneficial social connections that are linked to health outcomes (Phelan et al., 2010). When people lack access and are unable to use and benefit from these important resources, health inequities take root and persist. One fundamental resource for improving the health of people with SMI is to provide everyone accessible and affordable high-quality health care. Universal health care access to all people with SMI is an important step for achieving equity in health care as it eliminates from the equation the economic barriers that prevent many from seeking and using medical care. Health care is a basic human right, and the ability to pay for health services should not play any role in the decisions to receive high-quality health care.

The ongoing effort to build behavioral health homes for people with SMI throughout the United States is a critical step toward ensuring this important goal (Fortuna et al., 2020). These national efforts need to continue so that the investments already made in building this important health care infrastructure can be sustained and flourish. Let's not repeat the mistakes from the past in transforming the care of people with SMI in the United States; we need to make sure we properly fund and support the creation of a robust network of community-based behavioral health homes throughout our nation. Federal and state legislations and partnerships with managed care companies are needed to solidify these important efforts and develop the financial mechanisms, reimbursement codes, payment schemes, incentives, and administrative supports to ensure these integrated models of care and

all the services embedded in these models, including care coordination activities and the health care manager workforce, are properly funded and reimbursed so that they become routine care for all people with SMI.

But as discussed in Chapter 6, better access and quality of health care are critical, yet they may not be enough to improve the physical health and reduce premature mortality in people with SMI (Druss et al., 2017). The existing evidence indicates that integrated models of care for people with SMI like behavioral health homes can improve access and quality of health care; however, these benefits in health care do not seem to translate into consistent improvements in objective health indicators (e.g., blood pressure, glucose levels, weight) linked to premature mortality in people with SMI (Fortuna et al., 2020). Emerging studies show that for integrated models of care to achieve these important health outcomes, they need to include a complex package of services and supports that proactively focus on cardiovascular health by combining pharmacological treatments with self-management and behavioral approaches tailored for people with SMI that explicitly target smoking cessation, physical activity, healthy dietary habits, and the management and control of blood pressure, cholesterol, and blood sugar levels (Daumit et al., 2020).

The jury is still out in identifying the best package of services that need to be included in integrated models of care to produce clinically meaningful and lasting health improvements in people with SMI. As a mental health services researcher and social work scholar, I would be remiss not to discuss some key recommendations for what I think is needed to move these areas of research and practice forward, particularly in areas that have tended to be ignored in the existing literature for improving the health of people with SMI (Firth et al., 2019; Liu et al., 2017). I think two critical things are needed to continue advancing this work.

First, more multisite randomized effectiveness trials that enroll large numbers of racially and ethnically diverse populations are greatly needed to examine the impact and generalizability of integrated models of care in these historically marginalized and understudied communities. Despite the fact that in the United States racial and ethnic minorities, particularly Blacks and in many areas of the country Latino/as, are overrepresented in the public mental health system and publicly funded safety-net clinics, these diverse populations are often absent from, excluded from, or seriously underrepresented in the trials examining the effectiveness of integrated models of care and other health interventions (e.g., smoking cessation treatments, healthy

lifestyle programs) for people with SMI (Cabassa et al., 2017; Cabassa et al., 2010). This is one of the main reasons for including the stories, voices, and descriptions of people like Carla, Miguel, Enrique, Mr. S, and the others represented in this book that are often excluded from the scientific literature.

Furthermore, almost no study has directly examined and reported the differential outcomes of these interventions in these diverse populations. In fact, there is serious silence and inattention in our research literature examining the health of people with SMI regarding issues of racial and ethnic diversity, institutionalized racism, and how cultural factors and structural forces shape the health of people with SMI. For example, in a systematic literature review of interventions that aimed to address the medical conditions and health-risk behaviors in people with SMI that included 108 studies published between January 2000 and June 2014, there is not a single mention of issues of race, ethnicity, racism, or culture (McGinty et al., 2015a). As we discussed in previous publications, "the exclusion of historically underserved communities in clinical trials creates serious blind spots not only in treatment science but in moving this science into practice" (Baumann & Cabassa, 2020). We need to develop the evidence on how to make these integrated models of care work for everyone and better understand the impact and potential benefits these models of care have in historically marginalized racial and ethnic communities.

Health equity requires inclusion and representation of and true partnerships and engagement with communities of color. A one-size-fits-all approach to improve the health of people with SMI could create more harm than good because this approach tends to ignore and obfuscate the unique needs, characteristics, circumstances, and social conditions that shape the lives and health of people with SMI, particularly those from historically marginalized communities. An equity lens forces us to ask about these unique differences and to explicitly consider and address the specific needs of these diverse communities.

The next generation of effectiveness trials testing health interventions for people with SMI in my opinion needs to reflect the realities, conditions, and diversity of the populations served in routine practice settings. We need to make sure these effectiveness trials put equity for these historically marginalized communities front and center by carefully examining and reporting the processes and outcomes of care in these populations. More granularity in our studies is needed to better examine and understand how these interventions work for whom and under which conditions. To

develop a robust, generalizable, and equitable science that can inform clinical practice in the public mental health system and safety-net clinics, we need to make sure our studies include, engage with, and partner with historically marginalized communities that are most in need of these health interventions and programs.

My second recommendation for advancing research in this area focuses on bringing research and practice closer together by making sure the interventions and programs being developed, tested, and eventually implemented can be used, embedded, and sustained in the public mental health system. Investment in how to best implement the interventions and programs that we know work and have shown in randomized effectiveness trials to improve the health and health care of people with SMI was another consistent recommendation put forward by many of the clinicians and researchers interviewed for this book. This recommendation was clearly captured by Mary Brunette's call for making sure that the health interventions that are being developed and studied for people with SMI are "very portable and something that can be used by lay staff." We want to make sure that the existing workforce providing care for this population can use and deploy these interventions and that they have the resources, training, supervision, and supports they need to deliver this care. As we learned from Dr. Brunette's work in Chapter 7, the versatility of technology-based and - assisted interventions can be harnessed to increase the reach and benefits of health interventions, like smoking cessation programs. We also need the necessary policies, regulations, and financial structures to support the implementation and sustainment of these interventions. No matter how well trained and supervised our clinicians are, if our current policies, regulations, and reimbursement schemes do not pay and provide the resources and infrastructure necessary for these interventions, nothing will be implemented and sustained.

Addressing these important concerns requires increased investments in implementation science. As discussed by Stephen Bartels during our conversation, "We need to figure out how to implement these things [referring to health interventions for people with SMI like In Shape], get these things out here, get them used. We know what works, but we can't get it done right." Implementation science is a field of study that focuses on examining how to get interventions, programs, and/or policies integrated and ultimately sustained in routine practice settings to improve the processes, quality, and outcomes of care (Palinkas & Soydan, 2012; Proctor et al., 2009).

A specific area within the implementation science field that is greatly needed for improving the health of people with SMI is to focus on developing, testing, and using the most robust, useful, and effective implementation strategies to support the deployment and implementation of integrated models of care throughout our public mental health system and safety-net health clinics.

Implementation strategies are planned actions designed to facilitate the integration of new interventions into specific routine practice settings like outpatient mental health clinics (Powell et al., 2012). These strategies are used "to plan, educate, finance, restructure, manage quality, and attend to the policy context to facilitate implementation" (Powell et al., 2012, p. 193). I like to think of implementation strategies as the interventions for our interventions; these are the set of activities, administrative operations, steps, resources, supports, knowledge, skills, collaborations, partnerships, and infrastructure needed for an organization to be able to deliver and ultimately integrate a new intervention or program, such as integrated models of care, into their routine operations. We can no longer rely on just publishing the results of great studies and providing one-time training to clinicians and then hoping that these complex, multifaceted integrated models of care that require fundamental changes in how care is delivered get implemented in routine practice settings without further supports and assistance. Change in any organization is hard and requires concerted and strategic efforts, resources, time, and support from all levels of the organization. What is needed are implementation studies that link specific implementation strategies to specific health interventions and then test their effectiveness in getting these interventions integrated into routine practice settings. These are studies that focus not only on testing whether an intervention works but also on testing and directly examining how to make the intervention work within a specific setting. Basically, they examine what are the things that need to happen in an organization so that they can successfully deliver the intervention as intended to achieve the intended processes and outcomes of care.

A great example of this type of implementation study is an ongoing clustered randomized trial (NCT03891368) that is testing the impact of two types of implementation strategies for In Shape in 48 mental health organizations across the United States (Aschbrenner et al., 2019). Each organization is being randomized to receive two different implementation strategies over an 18-month period to support the implementation of In Shape. The goal is to rigorously test which implementation strategy works best in supporting the implementation of this health intervention in these organizations. In this

trial, every organization receives a 4-day in-person training on the In Shape model as well as expert supervision for the first 6 months of the study. One set of organizations will be randomized to receive a set of technical assistance activities that include four scheduled conference calls and the option for sites in this condition to request additional calls as needed throughout the 18 months after receiving the In Shape training. These technical assistance calls are tailored to each site and will use a structured approach to discuss key activities and issues related to the implementation of In Shape, including participant engagement, integration of the program within the agency, and the role of the health mentor, among others. Technical assistance is a common approach used to implement complex health interventions.

The other set of organizations will be randomized to receive a more intensive implementation strategy that uses a virtual learning collaborative approach. This approach employs quality improvement techniques such as setting goals and conducting small tests using the Plan-Do-Study-Act cycles, and sharing data as well as successes and failures with a community of organizations going through the same process (Ayers et al., 2005). Organizations in this condition will be required to attend monthly 90-minute web-based sessions to support their implementation of In Shape. The goal of this condition is to create a peer-to-peer community of organizations that support each other throughout the implementation process. To continue to move the field forward, we need more investments in these types of implementation trials to help identify the most robust and feasible strategies that can help us achieve the goal of making sure integrated models of care for people with SMI are the norm, not the exception, in our system of care.

Move Beyond the Clinic Walls

Efforts to improve the health of people with SMI need to move beyond focusing on individual behaviors and personal agency and carefully consider and examine the social conditions that impact the health and health care of this population. We need to raise our analytical and intervention gaze to consider that health behaviors do not happen in a vacuum but instead are greatly influenced by the structural forces and social conditions that shape people's lives, circumstances, and choices. As discussed in Chapter 2, the choices people with SMI make regarding their diets and physical activity; whether

they smoke or use substances; and whether they seek, use, and engage in medical care are influenced by their environment.

To improve the health of people with SMI, we need to not only integrate health and mental health care but also pay attention to the social conditions that shape people's health and well-being. Many people with SMI live in poverty, yet people's economic, structural, and social barriers are rarely considered in the development, testing, and deployment of health interventions for this population. How can we help people with SMI improve their dietary habits if they live in places where fresh fruits and vegetables are unavailable and unaffordable, if their neighborhoods have more fast-food establishments than grocery stores, and if food insecurity is a daily struggle? How can we continue to ignore the fact that many people with SMI are unemployed and living with extremely limited incomes, mostly relying on Supplemental Security Income or Social Security Disability Insurance to survive, forcing many to make difficult decisions as to whether to use their monthly resources to eat, pay rent and utilities, or pay for their medications and medical treatments? Without intervening in improving the social conditions of people with SMI, we will not be able to truly flatten the mortality curve in this population.

These complex problems have no magic solution, and there is no specific intervention or program I can point to at this time that is using a multilevel community approach to reduce health inequities in people with SMI. Improving the social conditions of people with SMI requires fundamental changes in how we view the health of this population and how we address issues beyond the clinic walls that go beyond health care, like increasing affordable and stable housing, improving food environments and neighborhood safety, and increasing education and stable employment opportunities. Multilevel community interventions and policies that target multiple social determinants of health at once, particularly those that help lift people out of poverty, are greatly needed. Dr. Vetta L. Thompson, a colleague from the Brown School at Washington University in St. Louis, whom I greatly admire for her dedication and work in eliminating health inequities recently wrote what I think encapsulates where our field needs to go: "To achieve equity, we must be willing to intervene directly on the social determinants and the practices and policies that sustain the systems of inequity" (Thompson, 2020, p. 41).

The recommendations discussed in this chapter may be difficult to implement and seem insurmountable given that they require fundamental

transformations in clinical practices and behavioral health and social policies, as well as investments in infrastructure, programs, and services. They require clinicians, administrators, policymakers, and advocates to realign how we approach, view, and provide treatments for the health of people with SMI within the health and mental health systems. These changes require a commitment to achieving health equity. But let us not forget and lose sight that these changes are possible.

Remember the experience of Miguel in Chapter 1 who was able to gain control of his diabetes and cholesterol levels with the support, encouragement, and resources provided by his health care manager using a culturally adapted intervention. Or recall the experience of Mr. S in Chapter 5 who described how he was able to break the cycles of unhealthy behaviors in unhealthy environments by engaging in a peer-led healthy lifestyle program delivered in his supportive housing program that brought this opportunity to his doorstep. And let us not forget about Marta's story from Chapter 7 and how a routine visit to her health care manager saved her life. Our failure to act can no longer be an excuse for not implementing the fundamental and pragmatic reforms that are needed to flatten the premature mortality curve. We know what is needed to end the unnecessary and preventable suffering and deaths of people with SMI. As my dad (*que en paz descanse*) used to say, "*hay que ponerle ganas, coño.*" What we need is the collective, social, and political will, *las ganas*, to end these deadly health inequities.

Notes

Chapter 1

1. To protect people's identity and confidentiality, I use fictitious names for all the people described in this book. I have also altered details such as place of birth, geographical location, age, and gender, among others, to ensure their anonymity. The information from these case studies comes from our different studies over the past 10 years and is a composite of different people.
2. SMRs are calculated by dividing the number of deaths in a study population, in this case people with schizophrenia, by the number of expected deaths adjusted for age- and sex-specific mortality rates in a standard population, in this case the general population. It serves as a measure for determining if the study population is at increased risk of dying compared to the standard population (Saha et al., 2007).

References

Alakeson, V., Frank, R. G., & Katz, R. E. (2010). Specialty care medical homes for people with severe, persistent mental disorders. *Health Affairs, 29*(5), 867–873. https://doi.org/10.1377/hlthaff.2010.0080

Alegria, M., Chatterji, P., Wells, K., Cao, Z., Chen, C. N., Takeuchi, D., Jackson, J., Meng, X. L. (2008). Disparity in depression treatment among racial and ethnic minority populations in the United States. *Psychiatric Services, 59*(11), 1264–1272. doi:10.1176/appi.ps.59.11.1264

Ali, M. K., Echouffo-Tcheugui, J., & Williamson, D. F. (2012). How effective were lifestyle interventions in real-world settings that were modeled on the Diabetes Prevention Program? *Health Affairs, 31*(1), 67–75. https://doi.org/10.1377/hlthaff.2011.1009

Allison, D. B., Newcomer, J. W., Dunn, A. L., Blumenthal, J. A., Fabricatore, A. N., Daumit, G. L., Cope, M. B., Riley, W. T., Vreeland, B. J. R., & Alpert, J. E. (2009). Obesity among those with mental disorders: A National Institute of Mental Health meeting report. *American Journal of Preventative Medicine, 36*(4), 341–350. https://doi.org/S0749-3797(09)00024-5[pii]10.1016/j.amepre.2008.11.020

American Diabetes Association, American Psychiatric Association, American Association of Clinical Endocrinologists, & North American Association for the Study of Obesity. (2004). Consensus development conference on antipsychotic drugs and obesity and diabetes. *Diabetes Care, 27*(2), 596–601. https://doi.org/10.2337/diacare.27.2.596

American Psychiatric Association. (2006). *Practice guideline for the treatment of patients with substance use disorders* (2nd ed.). https://psychiatryonline.org/pb/assets/raw/sitewide/practice_guidelines/guidelines/substanceuse.pdf

Aschbrenner, K., Carpenter-Song, E., Mueser, K., Kinney, A., Pratt, S., & Bartels, S. (2013). A qualitative study of social facilitators and barriers to health behavior change among persons with serious mental illness. *Community Mental Health Journal, 49*(2), 207–212. https://doi.org/10.1007/s10597-012-9552-8

Aschbrenner, K. A., Naslund, J. A., Gorin, A. A., Mueser, K. T., Browne, J., Wolfe, R. S., Xie, H., & Bartels, S. J. (2022). Group lifestyle intervention with mobile health for young adults with serious mental illness: A randomized controlled trial. *Psychiatric Services, 73*(2), 141–148. https://doi.org/10.1176/appi.ps.202100047

Aschbrenner, K. A., Pratt, S. I., Bond, G. R., Zubkoff, L., Naslund, J. A., Jue, K., Williams, G., Kinney, A., Cohen, M. J., Godfrey, M. M., & Bartels, S. J. (2019). A virtual learning collaborative to implement health promotion in routine mental health settings: Protocol for a cluster randomized trial. *Contemporary Clinical Trials, 84*, a105816. https://doi.org/10.1016/j.cct.2019.105816

Ayers, L. R., Beyea, S. C., Godfrey, M. M., Harper, D. C., Nelson, E. C., & Batalden, P. B. (2005). Quality improvement learning collaboratives. *Quality Management in Health Care, 14*(4), 234–247. https://doi.org/10.1097/00019514-200510000-00010

Barker, P. R., Manderscheid, R. W., Hendershot, G. E., Jack S. S., Schoenborn, C. A., & Goldstrom I. (1992). Serious mental illness and disability in the adult household population: United States, 1989. *Advanced Data, 1992*(218), 1–11. https://doi.org/10.1037/e608882007-001

Bartels, S. J., Aschbrenner, K. A., Pratt, S. I., Naslund, J. A., Scherer, E. A., Zubkoff, L., Cohen, M. J., Williams, G. W., Wolfe, R. S., Jue, K., & Brunette, M. F. (2018). Implementation of a lifestyle intervention for people with serious mental illness in state-funded mental health centers. *Psychiatric Services, 69*(6), 664–670. https://doi.org/10.1176/appi.ps.201700368

Bartels, S. J., Baggett, T., Freudenreich, O., & Bird, B. L. (2020). COVID-19 emergency reforms in Massachusetts to support behavioral health care and reduce mortality of people with serious mental illness. *Psychiatric Services, 71*(10), 1078–1081. https://www.bhchp.org/sites/default/files/publications/Bartels%20Baggett%20Freudenreich%20et%20al%202020.pdf

Bartels, S. J., & Desilets, R. A. (2012). *Health promotion programs for persons with serious mental illness: What works? A systematic review and analysis of the evidence base in published research literature on exercise and nutrition programs.* https://chess.wisc.edu/niatx/pdf/wicollaborative/HealthPromoSMI.pdf

Bartels, S. J., Pratt, S. I., Aschbrenner, K. A., Barre, L. K., Jue, K., Wolfe, R. S., Xie, H., McHugo, G., Santos, M., Williams, G. E., Naslund, J. A., & Mueser, K. T. (2013). Clinically significant improved fitness and weight loss among overweight persons with serious mental illness. *Psychiatric Services, 64*(8), 729–736. https://doi.org/10.1176/appi.ps.003622012

Bartels, S. J., Pratt, S. I., Aschbrenner, K. A., Barre, L. K., Naslund, J. A., Wolfe, R., Haiyi Xie, H., McHugo, G. J., Jimenez, D. E., Jue, K., Feldman, J., & Bird, B. L. (2015). Pragmatic replication trial of health promotion coaching for obesity in serious mental illness and maintenance of outcomes. *American Journal of Psychiatry, 172*(4), 344–352. https://doi.org/10.1176/appi.ajp.2014.14030357

Baumann, A. A., & Cabassa, L. J. (2020). Reframing implementation science to address inequities in healthcare delivery. *BMC Health Services Research, 20*(1), 190. https://doi.org/10.1186/s12913-020-4975-3

Bellack, A. S., Bennett, M. E., Gearon, J. S., Brown, C. H., & Yang, Y. (2006). A randomized clinical trial of a new behavioral treatment for drug abuse in people with severe and persistent mental illness. *Archives of General Psychiatry, 63*(4), 426–432. https://doi.org/10.1001/archpsyc.63.4.426

Berenson, A. (2006a, December 21). Disparity emerges in Lilly data on schizophrenia drug. *New York Times.* https://www.nytimes.com/2006/12/18/business/18drug.html

Berenson, A. (2006b, December 18). Drug files who maker promoted unapproved use. *New York Times.* https://www.nytimes.com/2006/12/18/business/18drug.html

Berenson, A. (2007, January 5). Lilly settles with 18,000 over Zyprexa. *New York Times.* https://www.nytimes.com/2007/01/05/business/05drug.html

Biswas, A., Oh, P. I., Faulkner, G. E., Bajaj, R. R., Silver, M. A., Mitchell, M. S., & Alter, D. A. (2015). Sedentary time and its association with risk for disease incidence, mortality, and hospitalization in adults: A systematic review and meta-analysis. *Annals of Internal Medicine, 162*(2), 123–132. https://doi.org/10.7326/M14-1651

Bochicchio, L., Stefancic, A., Gurdak, K., Swarbrick, M., & Cabassa, L. J. (2019). "We're all in this together": Peer-specialist contributions to a healthy lifestyle intervention for people with serious mental illness. *Administration of Policy in Mental Health and Mental Health Services Research, 46*(3), 298–310. https://doi.org/10.1007/s10488-018-0914-6

Borba, C. P., DePadilla, L., McCarty, F. A., von Esenwein, S. A., Druss, B. G., & Sterk, C. E. (2012). A qualitative study examining the perceived barriers and facilitators to medical healthcare services among women with a serious mental illness. *Womens Health Issues*, 22(2), e217–e224. https://doi.org/10.1016/j.whi.2011.10.001

Bradford, D. W., Kim, M. M., Braxton, L. E., Marx, C. E., Butterfield, M., & Elbogen, E. B. (2008). Access to medical care among persons with psychotic and major affective disorders. *Psychiatric Services*, 59(8), 847–852. https://doi.org/10.1176/ps.2008.59.8.847

Brunette, M. F., Ferron, J. C., McGurk, S. R., Williams, J. M., Harrington, A., Devitt, T., & Xie, H. (2020). Brief, web-based interventions to motivate smokers with schizophrenia: Randomized trial. *Journal of Medical Internet Research Mental Health*, 7(2), e16524. https://doi.org10.2196/16524

Cabassa, L. J. (2016). Implementation science: Why it matters for the future of social work. *Journal of Social Work Education*, 52(Suppl 1), S38–S50. https://doi.org/10.1080/10437797.2016.1174648

Cabassa, L. J., Camacho, D., Velez-Grau, C. M., & Stefancic, A. (2017). Peer-based health interventions for people with serious mental illness: A systematic literature review. *Journal of Psychiatric Research*, 84, 80–89. https://doi.org/10.1016/j.jpsychires.2016.09.021

Cabassa, L. J., Druss, B., Wang, Y., & Lewis-Fernandez, R. (2011). Collaborative planning approach to inform the implementation of a healthcare manager intervention for Hispanics with serious mental illness: A study protocol. *Implement Science*, 6, 80. https://doi.org/1748-5908-6-80

Cabassa, L. J., Ezell, J. M., & Lewis-Fernandez, R. (2010). Lifestyle interventions for adults with serious mental illness: A systematic literature review. *Psychiatric Services*, 61(8), 774–782. https://doi.org/10.1176/ps.2010.61.8.774

Cabassa, L. J., Gomes, A. P., Meyreles, Q., Capitelli, L., Younge, R., Dragatsi, D., Alvarez, J., Manrique, Y., & Lewis-Fernandez, R. (2014). Using the collaborative intervention planning framework to adapt a health-care manager intervention to a new population and provider group to improve the health of people with serious mental illness. *Implementation Science*, 9, a178. https://doi.org/10.1186/s13012-014-0178-9

Cabassa, L. J., Gomes, A. P., Meyreles, Q., Capitelli, L., Younge, R., Dragatsi, D., Alvarez, J., Nicasio, A., Druss, B., & Lewis-Fernandez, R. (2014). Primary health care experiences of Hispanics with serious mental illness: A mixed-methods study. *Administration and Policy in Mental Health and Mental Health Service Research*, 41(6), 724–736. https://doi.org/10.1007/s10488-013-0524-2

Cabassa, L. J., Hansen, M. C., Palinkas, L. A., & Ell, K. (2008). Azucar y nervios: Explanatory models and treatment experiences of Hispanics with diabetes and depression. *Social Science Medicine*, 66(12), 2413–2424. https://doi.org/10.1016/j.socscimed.2008.01.054

Cabassa, L. J., Manrique, Y., Meyreles, Q., Camacho, D., Capitelli, L., Younge, R., Dragatsi, D., Alvarez, J., & Lewis-Fernandez, R. (2016). Bridges to better health and wellness: An adapted health care manager intervention for Hispanics with serious mental illness. *Administration of Policy in Mental Health and Mental Health Services Research*, 45, 163–173. https://doi.org/10.1007/s10488-016-0781-y

Cabassa, L. J., Manrique, Y., Meyreles, Q., Capitelli, L., Younge, R., Dragatsi, D., Alvarez, J., & Lewis-Fernandez, R. (2019). "Treated me . . . like I was family": Qualitative evaluation of a culturally-adapted health care manager intervention for Latinos with serious mental illness and at risk for cardiovascular disease. *Transcultural Psychiatry*, 56(6), 1218–1236. https://doi.org/10.1177/1363461518808616

Cabassa, L. J., Parcesepe, A., Nicasio, A., Baxter, E., Tsemberis, S., & Lewis-Fernandez, R. (2013). Health and wellness photovoice project: Engaging consumers with serious mental illness in health care interventions. *Qualitative Health Research, 23*(5), 618–630. https://doi.org/10.1177/1049732312470872

Cabassa, L. J., Siantz, E., Nicasio, A., Guarnaccia, P., & Lewis-Fernandez, R. (2014). Contextual factors in the health of people with serious mental illness. *Qualitative Health Research, 24*(8), 1126–1137. https://doi.org/10.1177/1049732314541681

Cabassa, L. J., Stefancic, A., Lewis-Fernandez, R., Luchsinger, J., Weinstein, L. C., Guo, S., Palinkas, L., Bochicchio, L., Wang, X, O'Hara K., Blady, M., Simiriglia, C., & Medina McCurdy, M. (2021). Main outcomes of a peer-led healthy lifestyle intervention for people with serious mental illness in supportive housing. *Psychiatric Services, 72*(5), 555–562. doi:10.1176/appi.ps.202000304

Cabassa, L. J., Stefancic, A., O'Hara, K., El-Bassel, N., Lewis-Fernandez, R., Luchsinger, J. A., Gates, L., Younge, R., Wall, M., Weinstein, L., & Palinkas, L. A. (2015). Peer-led healthy lifestyle program in supportive housing: Study protocol for a randomized controlled trial. *Trials, 16*, a388. https://doi.org/10.1186/s13063-015-0902-z

Cabassa, L. J., Stefancic, A., Wang, X., Guo, S., Lu, N. Y., & Weatherly, C. (2020). Correlates of physical activity and cardiorespiratory fitness in racially and ethnically diverse people with serious mental illness in supportive housing. *Community Mental Health Journal, 56*(6), 1139–1152. https://doi.org10.1007/s10597-020-00610-x

Callaghan, R. C., Veldhuizen, S., Jeysingh, T., Orlan, C., Graham, C., Kakouris, G., Remington, G., & Gatley, J. (2014). Patterns of tobacco-related mortality among individuals diagnosed with schizophrenia, bipolar disorder, or depression. *Journal Psychiatric Research, 48*(1), 102–110. https://doi.org/10.1016/j.jpsychires.2013.09.014

Campion, J., Checinski, K., Nurse, J., & McNeill, A. (2008). Smoking by people with mental illness and benefits of smoke-free mental health services. *Advances in Psychiatric Treatment, 14*, 217–228. https://doi.org/10.1192/apt.bp.108.005710

Cannuscio, C. C., Weiss, E. E., & Asch, D. A. (2010). The contribution of urban foodways to health disparities. *Journal of Urban Health, 87*(3), 381–393. https://doi.org/10.1007/s11524-010-9441-9

Carter, R. (2010). *Within our reach: Ending the mental health crisis.* Rodale.

Castillo, E. G., Pincus, H. A., Smith, T. E., Miller, G., & Fish, D. G. (2017). New York State Medicaid reforms: Opportunities and challenges to improve the health of those with serious mental illness. *Journal of Health Care for the Poor and Underserved, 28*(3), 839–852. doi:10.1353/hpu.2017.0081

Centers for Disease Control and Prevention. (2017a). *Basic information about breast cancer.* https://www.cdc.gov/cancer/breast/basic_info/index.htm

Centers for Disease Control and Prevention. (2017b). *Early release of selected estimates based on data from the January–March 2017 National Health Interview Survey.* https://www.cdc.gov/nchs/data/nhis/earlyrelease/Earlyrelease201709_07.pdf

Centers for Disease Control and Prevention. (2017c). *What is diabetes?* https://www.cdc.gov/diabetes/basics/diabetes.html

Chen, L. S., Baker, T., Brownson, R. C., Carney, R. M., Jorenby, D., Hartz, S., Smock, N., Johnson, M., Ziedonis, D., & Bierut, L. J. (2017). Smoking cessation and electronic cigarettes in community mental health centers: Patient and provider perspectives. *Community Mental Health Journal, 53*(6), 695–702. https://doi.org10.1007/s10597-016-0065-8

Chinman, M., George, P., Dougherty, R. H., Daniels, A. S., Ghose, S. S., Swift, A., & Delphin-Rittmon, M. E. (2014). Peer support services for individuals with serious mental illnesses: Assessing the evidence. *Psychiatric Services, 65*(4), 429–441. https://doi.org/10.1176/appi.ps.201300244

Chochinov, H. M., Martens, P. J., Prior, H. J., Fransoo, R., & Burland, E. (2009). Does a diagnosis of schizophrenia reduce rates of mammography screening? A Manitoba population-based study. *Schizophrenia Research, 113*, 95–100. https://doi.org/10.1016/j.schres.2009.04.022

Chwastiak, L., Vanderlip, E., & Katon, W. (2014). Treating complexity: Collaborative care for multiple chronic conditions. *International Review of Psychiatry, 26*(6), 638–647. https://doi.org/10.3109/09540261.2014.969689

Colton, C. W., & Manderscheid, R. W. (2006). Congruencies in increased mortality rates, years of potential life lost, and causes of death among public mental health clients in eight states. *Preventing Chronic Disease, 3*(2), A42. https://www.cdc.gov/pcd/issues/2006/apr/05_0180.htm

Cook, J. A. (2011). Peer-delivered wellness recovery services: From evidence to widespread implementation. *Psychiatric Rehabilitation Journal, 35*(2), 87–89. https://doi.org/10.2975/35.2.2011.87.89

Correll, C. U., Joffe, B. I., Rosen, L. M., Sullivan, T. B., & Joffe, R. T. (2015). Cardiovascular and cerebrovascular risk factors and events associated with second-generation antipsychotic compared to antidepressant use in a non-elderly adult sample: Results from a claims-based inception cohort study. *World Psychiatry, 14*(1), 56–63. https://doi.org/10.1002/wps.20187

Correll, C. U., Manu, P., Olshanskiy, V., Napolitano, B., Kane, J. M., & Malhotra, A. K. (2009). Cardiometabolic risk of second-generation antipsychotic medications during first-time use in children and adolescents. *JAMA, 302*(16), 1765–1773. https://doi.org/10.1001/jama.2009.1549

Correll, C. U., Robinson, D. G., Schooler, N. R., Brunette, M. F., Mueser, K. T., Rosenheck, R. A., Marcy, P., Addington, J., Estroff, S. E., Robinson, J., Penn, D. L., Azrin, S., Goldstein, A., Severe, J., Heinssen, R., & Kane, J. M. (2014). Cardiometabolic risk in patients with first-episode schizophrenia spectrum disorders: Baseline results from the RAISE-ETP study. *JAMA Psychiatry, 71*(12), 1350–1363. https://doi.org/10.1001/jamapsychiatry.2014.1314

Correll, C. U., Rubio, J. M., & Kane, J. M. (2018). What is the risk-benefit ratio of long-term antipsychotic treatment in people with schizophrenia? *World Psychiatry, 17*(2), 149–160. https://doi.org/10.1002/wps.20516

Curtis, J., Watkins, A., Rosenbaum, S., Teasdale, S., Kalucy, M., Samaras, K., & Ward, P. B. (2016). Evaluating an individualized lifestyle and life skills intervention to prevent antipsychotic-induced weight gain in first-episode psychosis. *Early Interventions in Psychiatry, 10*(3), 267–276. https://doi.org/10.1111/eip.12230

Das, S., & Prochaska, J. J. (2017). Innovative approaches to support smoking cessation for individuals with mental illness and co-occurring substance use disorders. *Expert Review Respiratory Medicine, 11*(10), 841–850. https://doi.org10.1080/17476348.2017.1361823

Daumit, G. L., Dalcin, A. T., Dickerson, F. B., Miller, E. R., Evins, A. E., Cather, C., Jerome, G., Young, D. R., Charleston, J. B., Gennusa, J. V., III., Goldsholl, S., Cook, C., Heller, A., McGinty, E. E., Crum, R. M., Appel, L. J., & Wang, N. Y. (2020). Effect

of a comprehensive cardiovascular risk reduction intervention in persons with serious mental illness: A randomized clinical trial. *JAMA Network Open, 3*(6), e207247. https://doi.org/10.1001/jamanetworkopen.2020.7247

Daumit, G. L., Dickerson, F. B., Wang, N. Y., Dalcin, A., Jerome, G. J., Anderson, C. A., Young, D. R., Frick, K. D., Yu, A., Gennusa, J. V., III, Oefinger, M., Crum, R. M., Charleston, J., Casagrande, S. S., Guallar, E., Goldberg, R. W., Campbell, L. M., & Appel, L. J. (2013). A behavioral weight-loss intervention in persons with serious mental illness. *New England Journal of Medicine, 368*, 1594–1602. https://doi.org/10.1056/NEJMoa1214530

Davidoff, F. (2009). Heterogeneity is not always noise: Lessons from improvement. *JAMA, 302*(23), 2580–2586. https://doi.org/10.1001/jama.2009.1845

Davidson, L., Chinman, M., Sells, D., & Rowe, M. (2006). Peer support among adults with serious mental illness: A report from the field. *Schizophrenia Bulletin, 32*(3), 443–450. https://doi.org/10.1093/sbj043[pii]10.1093/schbul/sbj043

De Hert, M., Cohen, D., Bobes, J., Cetkovich-Bakmas, M., Leucht, S., Ndetei, D. M., Newcomer, J. W., Uwakwe, R., Asai, I., Möller, H.-J., Gautam, S., Detraux, J., & Correll, C. U. (2011). Physical illness in patients with severe mental disorders. II. Barriers to care, monitoring and treatment guidelines, plus recommendations at the system and individual level. *World Psychiatry, 10*(2), 138–151. https://doi.org/10.1002/j.2051-5545.2011.tb00036.x

De Hert, M., Correll, C. U., Bobes, J., Cetkovich-Bakmas, M., Cohen, D., Asai, I., Detraux J., Gautam, S., Möller, H.-J., Ndetei, D. M., Newcomer, J. W., Uwakwe, R., & Leucht, S. (2011). Physical illness in patients with severe mental disorders. I. Prevalence, impact of medications and disparities in health care. *World Psychiatry, 10*(1), 52–77. https://doi.org/10.1002/j.2051-5545.2011.tb00014.x

De Hert, M., Dekker, J. M., Wood, D., Kahl, K. G., Holt, R. I., & Moller, H. J. (2009). Cardiovascular disease and diabetes in people with severe mental illness position statement from the European Psychiatric Association (EPA), supported by the European Association for the Study of Diabetes (EASD) and the European Society of Cardiology (ESC). *European Psychiatry, 24*(6), 412–424. https://doi.org/10.1016/j.eurpsy.2009.01.005

De Hert, M., Detraux, J., van Winkel, R., Yu, W., & Correll, C. U. (2011). Metabolic and cardiovascular adverse effects associated with antipsychotic drugs. *National Review of Endocrinology, 8*(2), 114–126. https://doi.org/10.1038/nrendo.2011.156

Depp, C. A., Bowie, C. R., Mausbach, B. T., Wolyniec, P., Thornquist, M. H., Luke, J. R., McGrath, J. A., Pulver, A. E., Patterson, T. L., & Harvey, P. D. (2015). Current smoking is associated with worse cognitive and adaptive functioning in serious mental illness. *Acta Psychiatrica Scandinavica, 131*(5), 333–341. https://doi.org10.1111/acps.12380

Diabetes Prevention Program Research Group, Knowler, W. C., Fowler, S. E., Hamman, R. F., Christophi, C. A., Hoffman, H. J., Brenneman, A. T., Brown-Friday, J. O., Goldberg, R., Venditti, E., & Nathan, D. M. (2009). 10-year follow-up of diabetes incidence and weight loss in the Diabetes Prevention Program outcomes study. *Lancet, 374*(9702), 1677–1686. https://doi.org/10.1016/S0140-6736(09)61457-4

Dickerson, F., Schroeder, J., Katsafanas, E., Khushalani, S., Origoni, A. E., Savage, C., Schweinfurth, L., Stallings, C. R., Sweeney, K., & Yolken, R. H. (2018). Cigarette smoking by patients with serious mental illness, 1999–2016: An increasing disparity. *Psychiatric Services, 69*(2), 147–153. https://doi.org10.1176/appi.ps.201700118

Dickerson, F., Stallings, C. R., Origoni, A. E., Vaughan, C., Khushalani, S., Schroeder, J., & Yolken, R. H. (2013). Cigarette smoking among persons with schizophrenia or bipolar disorder in routine clinical settings, 1999–2011. *Psychiatric Services, 64*(1), 44–50. https://doi.org10.1176/appi.ps.201200143

Dipasquale, S., Pariante, C. M., Dazzan, P., Aguglia, E., McGuire, P., & Mondelli, V. (2013). The dietary pattern of patients with schizophrenia: A systematic review. *Journal of Psychiatric Research, 47*(2), 197–207. https://doi.org/10.1016/j.jpsychires.2012.10.005

Dittmer, J. (2009). *The good doctors: The Medical Committee for Human Rights and the struggles for social justice in health care.* Bloomsbury Press.

Dixon-Woods, L., Bosk, C. L., Aveling, E. L., Goeschel, C. A., & Pronvost, P. J. (2011). Explaining Michigan: Developing an ex post theory of a quality improvement program. *Milbank Quarterly, 89*(2), 167–205. https://doi.org/10.1111/j.1468-0009.2011.00625.x

Druss, B. G., Bradford, W. D., Rosenheck, R. A., Radford, M. J., & Krumholz, H. M. (2001). Quality of medical care and excess mortality in older patients with mental disorders. *Archives of General Psychiatry, 58*(6), 565–572. https://doi.org/10.1001/archpsyc.58.6.565

Druss, B. G., Marcus, S. C., Campbell, J., Cuffel, B., Harnett, J., Ingoglia, C., & Mauer, B. (2008). Medical services for clients in community mental health centers: Results from a national survey. *Psychiatric Services, 59*(8), 917–920. https://doi.org/10.1176/ps.2008.59.8.917

Druss, B. G., von Esenwein, S. A., Compton, M. T., Rask, K. J., Zhao, L., & Parker, R. M. (2010). A randomized trial of medical care management for community mental health settings: The primary care access, referral, and evaluation (PCARE) study. *American Journal of Psychiatry, 167*(2), 151–159. https://doi.org/10.1176/appi.ajp.2009.09050691

Druss, B. G., von Esenwein, S. A., Glick, G. E., Deubler, E., Lally, C., Ward, M. C., & Rask, K. J. (2017). Randomized trial of an integrated behavioral health home: The health outcomes management and evaluation (HOME) study. *American Journal of Psychiatry, 174*(3), 246–255. https://doi.org/10.1176/appi.ajp.2016.16050507

Druss, B. G., Zhao, L., Von Esenwein, S., Morrato, E. H., & Marcus, S. C. (2011). Understanding excess mortality in persons with mental illness: 17-year follow up of a nationally representative US survey. *Medical Care, 49*(6), 599–604. doi:10.1097/MLR.0b013e31820bf86e

Ell, K., Katon, W., Cabassa, L. J., Xie, B., Lee, P. J., Kapetanovic, S., & Guterman, J. (2009). Depression and diabetes among low-income Hispanics: Design elements of a socioculturally adapted collaborative care model randomized controlled trial. *International Journal of Psychiatry Medicine, 39*(2), 113–132.

Escobar, J. I., Golding, J. M., Hough, R. L., Karno, M., Burnam, M. A., & Wells, K. B. (1987). Somatization in the community: Relationship to disability and use of services. *American Journal of Public Health, 77*(7), 837–840. https://doi.org/10.2105/ajph.77.7.837

Evins, A. E., Cather, C., & Laffer, A. (2015). Treatment of tobacco use disorders in smokers with serious mental illness: Toward clinical best practices. *Harvard Review of Psychiatry, 23*(2), 90–98. https://doi.org10.1097/HRP.0000000000000063

Ezell, J. M., Siantz, E., & Cabassa, L. J. (2013). Contours of usual care: Meeting the medical needs of diverse people with serious mental illness. *Journal of Health Care for the Poor and Underserved, 24*(4), 1552–1573. https://doi.org/10.1353/hpu.2013.0158

Farmer, P. (2013). Reimagining accompaniment: A doctor's tribute to Gustavo Gutierrez. In M. Griffin & J. Block Weiss (Eds.), *In the company of the poor: Conversations with Dr. Paul Farmer and Fr. Gustavo Gutierrez* (pp. 15–25). Orbis Book.

Faulkner, G., Cohn, T., & Remington, G. (2006). Validation of a physical activity assessment tool for individuals with schizophrenia. *Schizophrenia Research, 82*(2–3), 225–231. https://doi.org/S0920-9964(05)00482-2 [pii]10.1016/j.schres.2005.10.020

Ferron, J. C., Brunette, M. F., He, X., Xie, H., McHugo, G. J., & Drake, R. E. (2011). Course of smoking and quit attempts among clients with co-occurring severe mental illness and substance use disorders. *Psychiatric Services, 62*(4), 353–359. https://doi.org10.1176/ps.62.4.pss6204_0353

Ferron, J. C., Brunette, M. F., McHugo, G. J., Devitt, T. S., Martin, W. M., & Drake, R. E. (2011). Developing a quit smoking website that is usable by people with severe mental illnesses. *Psychiatric Rehabilitation Journal, 35*(2), 111–116. https://doi.org10.2975/35.2.2011.111.116

Firth, J., Siddiqi, N., Koyanagi, A., Siskind, D., Rosenbaum, S., Galletly, C., Allan, S., Caneo, C., Carney, R., Carvalho, A. F., Chatterton, M. L., Correll, C. U., Curtis, J., Gaughran, F., Heald, A., Hoare, E., Jackson, S. E., Kisely, S. Lovell, K., . . . Stubbs, B. (2019). The Lancet Psychiatry Commission: A blueprint for protecting physical health in people with mental illness. *Lancet Psychiatry, 6*(8), 675–712. https://doi.org/10.1016/S2215-0366(19)30132-4

Fortuna, K. L., DiMilia, P. R., Lohman, M. C., Cotton, B. P., Cummings, J. R., Bartels, S. J., Batsis, J. A., & Pratt, S. I. (2020). Systematic review of the impact of behavioral health homes on cardiometabolic risk factors for adults with serious mental illness. *Psychiatric Services, 71*(1), 57–74. https://doi.org/10.1176/appi.ps.201800563

Gates, J., Killackey, E., Phillips, L., & Alvarez-Jimenez, M. (2015). Mental health starts with physical health: Current status and future directions of non-pharmacological interventions to improve physical health in first-episode psychosis. *Lancet Psychiatry, 2*(8), 726–742. https://doi.org/10.1016/S2215-0366(15)00213-8

Gawande, A. (2020). We can solve the coronavirus-test mess now—If we want to. *New Yorker.* https://www.newyorker.com/science/medical-dispatch/we-can-solve-the-coronavirus-test-mess-now-if-we-want-to

Gentile, S. (2006). Long-term treatment with atypical antipsychotics and the risk of weight gain: A literature analysis. *Drug Safety, 29*(4), 303–319. https://doi.org/10.2165/00002018-200629040-00002

Gilbody, S., Peckham, E., Bailey, D., Arundel, C., Heron, P., Crosland, S., Fairhurst, C., Hewitt, C., Li, J., Parrott, S., Bradshaw, T., Horspool, M., Hughes, E., Hughes, T., Ker, S., Leahy, M., McCloud, T., Osborn, D., Reilly, J., Steare, T., & Vickers, C. (2019). Smoking cessation for people with severe mental illness (SCIMITAR+): A pragmatic randomised controlled trial. *Lancet Psychiatry, 6*(5), 379–390. https://doi.org10.1016/S2215-0366(19)30047-1

Handley, M., MacGregor, K., Schillinger, D., Sharifi, C., Wong, S., & Bodenheimer T. (2006). Using action plans to help primary care patients adopt healthy behaviors: A descriptive study. *Journal of the American Board of Family Medicine, 19,* 224–231. https://doi.org/10.3122/jabfm.19.3.224

Hawes, M. R., Danforth, M. L., Jacquelyn Perez-Flores, N., Bochicchio, L., Tuda, D., Stefancic, A., & Cabassa, L. J. (2022). Learning, doing and sticking with it: A qualitative study on achieving clinically significant reduction in cardiovascular disease risk in a healthy lifestyle intervention for people with serious mental illness. *Health and Social Care in the Community, 30*(5), e2989–e2999. https://doi.org/10.1111/hsc.13744

Henwood, B. F., Cabassa, L. J., Craig, C. M., & Padgett, D. K. (2013). Permanent supportive housing: Addressing homelessness and health disparities? *American Journal of Public Health, 103*(S2), S188–S192. https://doi.org/10.2105/AJPH.2013.301490

Henwood, B. F., Weinstein, L. C., & Tsemberis, S. (2011). Creating a medical home for homeless persons with serious mental illness. *Psychiatric Services, 62*(5), 561–562. https://doi.org/10.1176/appi.ps.62.5.561

Hjorthoj, C., Ostergaard, M. L., Benros, M. E., Toftdahl, N. G., Erlangsen, A., Andersen, J. T., & Nordentoft, M. (2015). Association between alcohol and substance use disorders and all-cause and cause-specific mortality in schizophrenia, bipolar disorder, and unipolar depression: A nationwide, prospective, register-based study. *Lancet Psychiatry, 2*(9), 801–808. https://doi.org/10.1016/S2215-0366(15)00207-2

Hogan, M. F. (2003). The President's New Freedom Commission: Recommendations to transform mental health care in America. *Psychiatric Services, 54*(11), 1467–1474. https://doi.org/10.1176/appi.ps.54.11.1467

Hooper, M. W., Napoles, A. M., & Perez-Stable, E. J. (2020). View point: COVOD-19 and racial/ethnic disparities. *JAMA, 323*(24), 2466–2467.

Institute of Medicine. (2003). *Unequal treatment: Confronting racial and ethnic disparities in health care.* https://pubmed.ncbi.nlm.nih.gov/25032386/

Institute of Medicine. (2006). *Improving the quality of health care for mental and substance use conditions* (Quality Chasm Series). https://www.ncbi.nlm.nih.gov/books/NBK19830/

Interdepartmental Serious Mental Illness Coordinating Committee. (2017). *The way forward: Federal action for a system that works for all people living with SMI and SED and their families and caregivers.* Substance Abuse and Mental Health Services Administration. https://store.samhsa.gov/product/PEP17-ISMICC-RTC

IphYs. (2018). *What is HeAl?* https://www.iphys.org.au/what-is-heal

Ivey, S. L., Scheffler, R., & Zazzali, J. L. (1998). Supply dynamics of the mental health workforce: Implications for health policy. *Milbank Quarterly, 76*(1), 25–58. https://doi.org/10.1111/1468-0009.00078

Janssen, E. M., McGinty, E. E., Azrin, S. T., Juliano-Bult, D., & Daumit, G. L. (2015). Review of the evidence: Prevalence of medical conditions in the United States population with serious mental illness. *General Hospital Psychiatry, 37*(3), 199–222. doi:10.1016/j.genhosppsych.2015.03.004

Jones, S., Howard, L., & Thornicroft, G. (2008). "Diagnostic overshadowing": Worse physical health care for people with mental illness. *Acta Psychiatrica Scandinavica, 118*(3), 169–171. https://doi.org/10.1111/j.1600-0447.2008.01211.x

Kessler, R. C., Barker, P. R., Colpe, L. J., Epstein, J. F., Gfroerer, J. C., Hiripi, E., Howes, M. J., Normand S. T., Manderscheid, R. W., Walters, E. E. & Zaslavsky, A. M. (2003). Screening for serious mental illness in the general population. *Archives of General Psychiatry, 60*(2), 184–189. https://doi.org/10.1001/archpsyc.60.2.184

Kilbourne, A. M., Greenwald, D. E., Bauer, M. S., Charns, M. P., & Yano, E. M. (2012). Mental health provider perspectives regarding integrated medical care for patients with serious mental illness. *Administration of Policy in Mental Health and Mental Health Services Research, 39*(6), 448–457. https://doi.org/10.1007/s10488-011-0365-9

Knowler, W. C., Barrett-Connor, E., Fowler, S. E., Hamman, R. F., Lachin, J. M., Walker, E. A., & Nathan, D. M. (2002). Reduction in the incidence of type 2 diabetes with lifestyle intervention or metformin. *New England Journal of Medicine, 346*(6), 393–403. https://doi.org/10.1056/NEJMoa012512

Kochanek, K. D., Arias, E., & Anderson, R. N. (2013). How did cause of death contribute to racial differences in life expectancy in the United States in 2010? *NCHS Data Brief,* (125), 1–8. https://pubmed.ncbi.nlm.nih.gov/24152376/

Kodama, S., Saito, K., Tanaka, S., Maki, M., Yachi, Y., Asumi, M., Sugawara, A., Totsuka, K., Shimano, H., Ohashi, Y., Yamada, N., & Sone, H. (2009). Cardiorespiratory fitness as a quantitative predictor of all-cause mortality and cardiovascular events in healthy men and women: A meta-analysis. *JAMA, 301*(19), 2024–2035. https://doi.org/10.1001/jama.2009.681

Koskinen, J., Lohonen, J., Koponen, H., Isohanni, M., & Miettunen, J. (2009). Prevalence of alcohol use disorders in schizophrenia—A systematic review and meta-analysis. *Acta Psychiatrica Scandinavica, 120*(2), 85–96. https://doi.org/10.1111/j.1600-0447.2009.01385.x

Kramer, M. K., Kriska, A. M., Venditti, E. M., Miller, R. G., Brooks, M. M., Burke, L. E., Siminerio, L. M., Solano, F. X., & Orchard, T. J. (2009). Translating the Diabetes Prevention Program: A comprehensive model for prevention training and program delivery. *American Journal of Preventative Medicine, 37*(6), 505–511. https://doi.org/10.1016/j.amepre.2009.07.020

Lasser, K., Boyd, J. W., Woolhandler, S., Himmelstein, D. U., McCormick, D., & Bor, D. H. (2000). Smoking and mental illness: A population-based prevalence study. *JAMA, 284*(20), 2606–2610. https://doi.org/10.1001/jama.284.20.2606

Lehrer, J. (2007, October 29). The listener: Brain & behaviors. *Seedmagazine.com.*

Lieberman, J. A., Stroup, T. S., McEvoy, J. P., Swartz, M. S., Rosenheck, R. A., Perkins, D. O., Keefe, R. S. E., Davis, S. M., Davis, C. E., Lebowitz, B. D., Severe, J. S., & Hsiao, J. K. (2005). Effectiveness of antipsychotic drugs in patients with chronic schizophrenia. *New England Journal Medicine, 353*(12), 1209–1223. https://doi.org/10.1056/NEJMoa051688

Liu, N. H., Daumit, G. L., Dua, T., Aquila, R., Charlson, F., Cuijpers, P., Druss, B., Dudek, K., Freeman, M., Fujii, C., Gaebel, W., Hegerl, U., Levav, I., Laursen, T. M., Ma, H., Maj, M., Medina-Mora, M. E., Nordentoft, M., Prabhakaran, D., . . . Saxena, S. (2017). Excess mortality in persons with severe mental disorders: A multilevel intervention framework and priorities for clinical practice, policy and research agendas. *World Psychiatry, 16*(1), 30–40. https://doi.org/10.1002/wps.20384

Lopez, S. R., & Guarnaccia, P. J. (2000). Cultural psychopathology: Uncovering the social world of mental illness. *Annual Review of Psychology, 51*, 571–598. https://doi.org/10.1146/annurev.psych.51.1.571

Malzberg, B. (1937). Mortality in involution melancholia. *American Journal of Psychiatry, 93*, 1231–1238. https://doi.org/10.1176/ajp.93.5.1231

Mangurian, C., Newcomer, J. W., Modlin, C., & Schillinger, D. (2016). Diabetes and cardiovascular care among people with severe mental illness: A literature review. *Journal of General Internal Medicine, 31*(9), 1083–1091. https://doi.org/10.1007/s11606-016-3712-4

Mangurian, C., Newcomer, J. W., Vittinghoff, E., Creasman, J. M., Knapp, P., Fuentes-Afflick, E., & Schillinger, D. (2015). Diabetes screening among underserved adults with severe mental illness who take antipsychotic medications. *JAMA Internal Medicine, 175*(12), 1977–1979. https://doi.org/10.1001/jamainternmed.2015.6098

Martens, P. J., Chochinov, H. M., Prior, H. J., Fransoo, R., & Burland, E. (2009). Are cervical cancer screening rates different for women with schizophrenia? A Manitoba

population-based study. *Schizophrenia Research, 113,* 101–106. https://doi.org/
10.1016/j.schres.2009.04.015

McGinty, E. E., Baller, J., Azrin, S. T., Juliano-Bult, D., & Daumit, G. L. (2015a).
Interventions to address medical conditions and health-risk behaviors among persons
with serious mental illness: A comprehensive review. *Schizophrenia Bulletin, 42*(1), 96–
124. https://doi.org/10.1093/schbul/sbv101

McGinty, E. E., Baller, J., Azrin, S. T., Juliano-Bult, D., & Daumit, G. L. (2015b). Quality
of medical care for persons with serious mental illness: A comprehensive review.
Schizophrenia Research, 165, 227–235. https://doi.org/10.1016/j.schres.2015.04.010

McGinty, E. E., Blasco-Colmenares, E., Zhang, Y., Dosreis, S. C., Ford, D. E., Steinwachs,
D. M., Guallar, E., & Daumit, G. L. (2012). Post-myocardial-infarction quality of
care among disabled Medicaid beneficiaries with and without serious mental illness.
General Hospital Psychiatry, 34(5), 493–499. https://doi.org/10.1016/j.genhospps
ych.2012.05.004

Mitchell, A. J., & Lord, O. (2010). Do deficits in cardiac care influence high mortality rates in schizophrenia? A systematic review and pooled analysis. *Journal of
Psychopharmacology, 24*(11), 69–80. https://doi.org/10.1177/1359786810382056

Mitchell, A. J., Vancampfort, D., De Hert, M., & Stubbs, B. (2015). Do people with mental
illness receive adequate smoking cessation advice? A systematic review and meta-
analysis. *General Hospital Psychiatry, 37*(1), 14–23. https://doi.org10.1016/j.genhospps
ych.2014.11.006

Mitchell, A. J., Vancampfort, D., Sweers, K., van Winkel, R., Yu, W., & De Hert, M. (2013).
Prevalence of metabolic syndrome and metabolic abnormalities in schizophrenia and
related disorders—A systematic review and meta-analysis. *Schizophrenia Bulletin,
39*(2), 306–318. https://doi.org/10.1093/schbul/sbr148

Murphy, K. A., Daumit, G. L., Stone, E., & McGinty, E. E. (2018). Physical health
outcomes and implementation of behavioural health homes: A comprehensive review.
International Review of Psychiatry, 30(6), 224–241. https://doi.org/10.1080/09540
261.2018.1555153

Nasrallah, H. A., Meyer, J. M., Goff, D. C., McEvoy, J. P., Davis, S. M., Stroup, T. S., &
Lieberman, J. A. (2006). Low rates of treatment for hypertension, dyslipidemia and di-
abetes in schizophrenia: Data from the CATIE schizophrenia trial sample at baseline.
Schizophrenia Research, 86(1–3), 15–22. https://doi.org/10.1016/j.schres.2006.06.026

National Association of State Mental Health Program Directors. (2014). *Enhancing the
peer provider workforce: Recruitment, supervision and retention.* https://www.nasm
hpd.org/content/enhancing-peer-provider-workforce-recruitment-supervision-and-
retention

National Council for Well Being. (2022). *Center of Excellence for Integrated Health
Solutions.* https://www.thenationalcouncil.org/program/center-of-excellence/

Nelson, G., & Laurier, W. (2010). Housing for people with serious mental illness: Approaches, evidence, and transformative change. *Journal of Sociology & Social
Welfare, 38*(4), 123–146. https://citeseerx.ist.psu.edu/viewdoc/download?doi=
10.1.1.854.2137&rep=rep1&type=pdf

Newcomer, J. W., & Haupt, D. W. (2006). The metabolic effects of antipsychotic
medications. *Canadian Journal of Psychiatry, 51*(8), 480–491. https://doi.org/10.1177/
070674370605100803

No mental health without physical health [Editorial]. (2011). *The Lancet, 377,* 611.

O'Brien, W. (2016). *Shawn Brown: A healthy balance.* https://projecthome.org/news/
shawn-brown-healthy-balance

Odegard, O. (1951). Mortality in Norwegian mental hospitals 1926–1941. *Acta Genetica
et Statistica Medica, 2*(2), 141–173. https://doi.org/10.1159/000150667

O'Hara, K., Stefancic, A., & Cabassa, L. J. (2017). Developing a peer-based healthy lifestyle
program for people with serious mental illness in supportive housing. *Translational
Behavioral Medicine, 7*(4), 793–803. https://doi.org/10.1007/s13142-016-0457-x

Olfson, M., Gerhard, T., Huang, C., Crystal, S., & Stroup, T. S. (2015). Premature mortality
among adults with schizophrenia in the United States. *JAMA Psychiatry, 72*(12), 1172–
1181. doi:10.1001/jamapsychiatry.2015.1737

Oluwoye, O., Monroe-DeVita, M., Burduli, E., Chwastiak, L., McPherson, S., McClellan,
J. M., & McDonell, M. G. (2019). Impact of tobacco, alcohol and cannabis use on treatment outcomes among patients experiencing first episode psychosis: Data from the
national RAISE-ETP study. *Early Interventions in Psychiatry, 13*(1), 142–146. https://
doi.org10.1111/eip.12542

Palinkas, L. A., & Soydan, H. (2012). New horizons of translational research and research
translation in social work. *Research on Social Work Practice, 22*(1), 85–92. https://doi.
org/10.1177/1049731511408738

Parks, J., Svendsen, D., Singer, P., & Foti, M. E. (2006). *Morbidity and mortality in people
with serious mental illness.* Report from the National Association of State Mental
Health Program Directors. http://www.oregonjobs.org/DHS/mentalhealth/wellness/
morbidity.pdf

Peckham, E., Brabyn, S., Cook, L., Tew, G., & Gilbody, S. (2017). Smoking cessation in severe mental ill health: What works? An updated systematic review and meta-analysis.
BMC Psychiatry, 17(1), a252. https://doi.org10.1186/s12888-017-1419-7

Pérez-Iglesias, R., Martínez-García, O., Pardo-Garcia, G., Amado, J. A., Garcia-Unzueta,
M. T., Tabares-Seisdedos, R., & Crespo-Facorro, B. (2014). Course of weight gain and
metabolic abnormalities in first treated episode of psychosis: The first year is a critical period for development of cardiovascular risk factors. *International Journal of
Neuropsychopharmacology, 17*(1), 41–51. https://doi.org/10.1017/S1461145713001053

Phelan, J. C., Link, B. G., & Tehranifar, P. (2010). Social conditions as fundamental causes
of health inequalities: Theory, evidence, and policy implications. *Journal of Health and
Social Behavior, 51*, S28–40. https://doi.org/10.1177/0022146510383498

Phutane, V. H., Tek, C., Chwastiak, L., Ratliff, J. C., Ozyuksel, B., Woods, S. W., & Srihari,
V. H. (2011). Cardiovascular risk in a first-episode psychosis sample: A "critical period"
for prevention? *Schizophrenia Research, 127*(1–3), 257–261. https://doi.org/10.1016/
j.schres.2010.12.008

Powell, B. J., McMillen, J. C., Proctor, E. K., Carpenter, C. R., Griffey, R. T., Bunger, A. C.,
Glass, J. E., & York, J. L. (2012). A compilation of strategies for implementing clinical
innovations in health and mental health. *Medical Care Research Review, 69*(2), 123–
157. https://doi.org/1077558711430690

Prochaska, J. J., Das, S., & Young-Wolff, K. C. (2017). Smoking, mental illness, and public
health. *Annual Review of Public Health, 38*, 165–185. https://doi.org10.1146/annurev-
publhealth-031816-044618

Prochaska, J. J., Fromont, S. C., Louie, A. K., Jacobs, M. H., & Hall, S. M. (2006). Training
in tobacco treatments in psychiatry: A national survey of psychiatry residency training
directors. *Academic Psychiatry, 30*(5), 372–378. https://doi.org/10.1176/appi.ap.30.5.372

Proctor, E. K., Landsverk, J., Aarons, G., Chambers, D., Glisson, C., & Mittman, B. (2009). Implementation research in mental health services: An emerging science with conceptual, methodological, and training challenges. *Administration of Policy in Mental Health and Mental Health Services Research, 36*(1), 24–34. https://doi.org/10.1007/s10 488-008-0197-4

Putz, J., Sapir, H., Macy, J., Lieberman, T. E., Forster, S. E., Reece, M., Mathes, K. A., Sheese, M., Andry, J. M., & Frasure, K. A. (2015). Integrated healthcare in a community-based mental health center: A longitudinal study of metabolic risk reduction. *Journal of Social Service Research, 41,* 584–598. https://doi.org/10.1080/01488376.2015.1072761

Rossen, L. M., Branum, A. M., Ahmad, F. B., Sutton, P., & Anderson, R. N. (2020). Excess deaths associated with COVID-19, by age and race and ethnicity—United States, January 26–October 3, 2020. *MMWR Morbidity and Mortal Weekly Report, 69*(42), 1522–1527. https://doi.org/10.15585/mmwr.mm6942e2

Saha, S., Chant, D., & McGrath, J. (2007). A systematic review of mortality in schizophrenia: Is the differential mortality gap worsening over time? *Archives of General Psychiatry, 64*(10), 1123–1131. doi:10.1001/archpsyc.64.10.1123

Sampson, U. K., Kaplan, R. M., Cooper, R. S., Diez Roux, A. V., Marks, J. S., Engelgau, M. M., Peprah E., Mishoe, H., Boulware, E., Felix, K. L., Califf, R. M., Flack, J. M., Cooper, L. A., Garcia, N., Henderson, J. A., Davidson, K. W., Krishnan J. A., Lewis, T. T., Sanchez, E. . . . Mensah, G. A. (2016). Reducing health inequities in the U.S.: Recommendations from the NHLBI's health inequities think tank meeting. *Journal of the American College of Cardiology, 68*(5), 517–524. doi:10.1016/j.jacc.2016.04.059

Scharf, D. M., Eberhart, N. K., Horvitz-Lennon, M., Beckman, R., Han, B., Lovejoy, S. L., Pincus, H. A., & Burnam, M. A. (2013). *Evaluation of the SAMHSA primary and Behavioral Care Integration (PBHCI) grant program: Final report.* https://pubmed.ncbi. nlm.nih.gov/28560076/

School of Pharmacy, University of California at San Francisco. (2022). *Rx for change.* https://rxforchange.ucsf.edu

Sharma, R., Gartner, C. E., & Hall, W. D. (2016). The challenge of reducing smoking in people with serious mental illness. *Lancet Respiratory Medicine, 4*(10), 835–844. https://doi.org10.1016/S2213-2600(16)30228-4

Sheals, K., Tombor, I., McNeill, A., & Shahab, L. (2016). A mixed-method systematic review and meta-analysis of mental health professionals' attitudes toward smoking and smoking cessation among people with mental illnesses. *Addiction, 111*(9), 1536–1553. https://doi.org10.1111/add.13387

Shiner, B., Whitley, R., Van Citters, A. D., Pratt, S. I., & Bartels, S. J. (2008). Learning what matters for patients: Qualitative evaluation of a health promotion program for those with serious mental illness. *Health Promotion International, 23*(3), 275–282. https:// doi.org/10.1093/heapro/dan018

Siantz, E., & Aranda, M. P. (2014). Chronic disease self-management interventions for adults with serious mental illness: A systematic review of the literature. *General Hospital Psychiatry, 36*(3), 233–244. https://doi.org/10.1016/j.genhosppsych.2014.01.014

Siru, R., Hulse, G. K., & Tait, R. J. (2009). Assessing motivation to quit smoking in people with mental illness: A review. *Addiction, 104*(5), 719–733. https://doi.org10.1111/ j.1360-0443.2009.02545.x

Srihari, V. H., Phutane, V. H., Ozkan, B., Chwastiak, L., Ratliff, J. C., Woods, S. W., & Tek, C. (2013). Cardiovascular mortality in schizophrenia: Defining a critical period for

prevention. *Schizophrenia Research, 146*(1–3), 64–68. https://doi.org/10.1016/j.sch res.2013.01.014

Stanhope, V., & Ashenberg Straussner, S. L. (Eds.). (2018). *Social work and integrated health care: From policy to practice and back.* Oxford University Press.

Stubbs, B., Firth, J., Berry, A., Schuch, F. B., Rosenbaum, S., Gaughran, F., Veronesse, N., Williams, J., Craig, T., Yung, A. R., & Vancampfort, D. (2016). How much physical activity do people with schizophrenia engage in? A systematic review, comparative meta-analysis and meta-regression. *Schizophrenia Research, 176*(2–3), 431–440. https://doi. org/10.1016/j.schres.2016.05.017

Stubbs, B., Vancampfort, D., Bobes, J., De Hert, M., & Mitchell, A. J. (2015). How can we promote smoking cessation in people with schizophrenia in practice? A clinical overview. *Acta Psychiatrica Scandinavica, 132*(2), 122–130. https://doi.org10.1111/acps.12412

Stubbs, B., Williams, J., Gaughran, F., & Craig, T. (2016). How sedentary are people with psychosis? A systematic review and meta-analysis. *Schizophrenia Research, 171*(1–3), 103–109. https://doi.org/10.1016/j.schres.2016.01.034

Substance Abuse and Mental Health Services Administration. (2017). *Mental and substance use disorders.* https://www.samhsa.gov/disorders

Substance Abuse and Mental Health Services Administration. (2021). *Key substance use and mental health indicators in the United States: Results from the 2020 National Survey on Drug Use and Health (HHS Publication No. PEP21-07-01-003, NSDUH Series H-56).* Rockville, MD: Center for Behavioral Health Statistics and Quality, Substance Abuse and Mental Health Services Administration. https://www.samhsa.gov/data

Substance Abuse and Mental Health Services Administration Center for Behavioral Health Statistics and Quality. (2014). *The NSDUH report: Substance use and mental health estimates from the 2013 National Survey on Drug Use and Health: Overview of findings.* https://pubmed.ncbi.nlm.nih.gov/27656739/

Tai, D. B. G., Shah, A., Doubeni, C. A., Sia, I. G., & Wieland, M. L. (2020). The disproportionate impact of COVID-19 on racial and ethnic minorities in the United States. *Clinical Infectious Diseases, 72*(4), 703–706. https://doi.org/10.1093/cid/ciaa815

Thompson, V. L. (2020). Inequity and the path to change. *Magazine of Washington University in St. Louis, 91*, 41.

Thornicroft, G. (2006). *Shunned: Discrimination against people with mental illness.* Oxford University Press.

Torniainen, M., Mittendorfer-Rutz, E., Tanskanen, A., Bjorkenstam, C., Suvisaari, J., Alexanderson, K., & Tiihonen, J. (2015). Antipsychotic treatment and mortality in schizophrenia. *Schizophrenia Bulletin, 41*(3), 656–663. https://doi.org/10.1093/schbul/ sbu164

U.S. Department of Health and Human Services. (2017). *Health and Human Services plan to reduce racial and ethnic health disparities.* https://minorityhealth.hhs.gov/omh/bro wse.aspx?lvl=2&lvlid=10

Van Citters, A. D., Pratt, S. I., Jue, K., Williams, G., Miller, P. T., Xie, H., & Bartels, S. J. (2010). A pilot evaluation of the In SHAPE individualized health promotion intervention for adults with mental illness. *Community Mental Health Journal, 46*(6), 540–552. https://doi.org/10.1007/s10597-009-9272-x

Vancampfort, D., Probst, M., Knapen, J., Carraro, A., & De Hert, M. (2012). Associations between sedentary behaviour and metabolic parameters in patients with schizophrenia. *Psychiatry Research, 200*(2–3), 73–78. https://doi.org/10.1016/j.psychres.2012.03.046

Vancampfort, D., Rosenbaum, S., Probst, M., Soundy, A., Mitchell, A. J., De Hert, M., & Stubbs, B. (2015). Promotion of cardiorespiratory fitness in schizophrenia: A clinical overview and metaanalysis. *Acta Psychiatrica Scandinavica, 132*, 131–143. https://doi.org/10.1111/acps.12407

Vancampfort, D., Wampers, M., Mitchell, A. J., Correll, C. U., De Herdt, A., Probst, M., & De Hert, M. (2013). A meta-analysis of cardio-metabolic abnormalities in drug naive, first-episode and multi-episode patients with schizophrenia versus general population controls. *World Psychiatry, 12*(3), 240–250. https://doi.org/10.1002/wps.20069

Vazin, R., McGinty, E. E., Dickerson, F., Dalcin, A., Goldsholl, S., Oefinger Enriquez, M., Jerome, G. J., Gennusa, J. V., III, & Daumit, G. L. (2016). Perceptions of strategies for successful weight loss in persons with serious mental illness participating in a behavioral weight loss intervention: A qualitative study. *Psychiatric Rehabilitation Journal, 39*(2), 137–146. https://doi.org/10.1037/prj0000182

Venditti, E. M., & Kramer, M. K. (2012). Necessary components for lifestyle modification interventions to reduce diabetes risk. *Current Diabetes Report, 12*(2), 138–146. https://doi.org/10.1007/s11892-012-0256-9

Verhaeghe, N., De Maeseneer, J., Maes, L., Van Heeringen, C., & Annemans, L. (2011). Effectiveness and cost-effectiveness of lifestyle interventions on physical activity and eating habits in persons with severe mental disorders: A systematic review. *International Journal of Behavioral Nutrition and Physical Activity, 8*, a28. https://doi.org/10.1186/1479-5868-8-28

Vermeulen, J., van Rooijen, G., Doedens, P., Numminen, E., van Tricht, M., & de Haan, L. (2017). Antipsychotic medication and long-term mortality risk in patients with schizophrenia: A systematic review and meta-analysis. *Psychological Medicine, 47*(13), 2217–2228. https://doi.org/10.1017/S0033291717000873

Vigo, D., Thornicroft, G., & Atun, R. (2016). Estimating the true global burden of mental illness. *Lancet Psychiatry, 3*(2), 171–178. doi:10.1016/S2215-0366(15)00505-2

Walker, E. R., McGee, R. E., & Druss, B. G. (2015). Mortality in mental disorders and global disease burden implications: A systematic review and meta-analysis. *JAMA Psychiatry, 72*(4), 334–341. doi:10.1001/jamapsychiatry.2014.2502

Weinstein, L. C., Stefancic, A., Cunningham, A. T., Hurley, K. E., Cabassa, L. J., & Wender, R. C. (2016). Cancer screening, prevention, and treatment in people with mental illness. *CA: A Cancer Journal for Clinicians, 66*(2), 134–151. doi:10.3322/caac.21334

West, D. S., Elaine, P. T., Bursac, Z., & Felix, H. C. (2008). Weight loss of Black, White, and Hispanic men and women in the diabetes prevention program. *Obesity, 16*, 1413–1420. https://doi.org/10.1038/oby.2008.224

Williams, D. R., Gonzalez, H. M., Neighbors, H., Nesse, R., Abelson, J. M., Sweetman, J., & Jackson, J. S. (2007). Prevalence and distribution of major depressive disorder in African Americans, Caribbean blacks, and non-Hispanic whites: results from the National Survey of American Life. *Archives of General Psychiatry, 64*(3), 305–315. doi:10.1001/archpsyc.64.3.305

World Health Organization. (2002). *30 minutes for a healthy life span* [Press release]. https://www.who.int/docstore/world-health-day/2002/euro_press.pdf

World Health Organization. (2017a). *Cancer* [Fact sheet]. http://www.who.int/mediacentre/factsheets/fs297/en/

World Health Organization. (2017b). *Diabetes* [Fact sheet]. http://www.who.int/mediacentre/factsheets/fs312/en/

World Health Organization. (2018). *Guidelines for the management of physical health conditions in adults with severe mental disorders.* https://apps.who.int/iris/bitstream/handle/10665/275718/9789241550383-eng.pdf

World Health Organization. (2021). *Cardiovascular diseases (CVDs) [Fact sheet].* https://www.who.int/news-room/fact-sheets/detail/cardiovascular-diseases-(cvds)

Yarborough, B. J., Stumbo, S. P., Yarborough, M. T., Young, T. J., & Green, C. A. (2016). Improving lifestyle interventions for people with serious mental illnesses: Qualitative results from the STRIDE study. *Psychiatric Rehabilitation Journal, 39*(1), 33–41. https://doi.org/10.1037/prj0000151

Zayas, L. H. (2015). *Forgotten citizens: Deportation, children, and the making of American exiles and orphans.* Oxford University Press.

Ziedonis, D., Hitsman, B., Beckham, J. C., Zvolensky, M., Adler, L. E., Audrain-McGovern, J., Breslau, N., Brown, R. A., George, T. P., Williams, J., Calhoun, P. S., & Riley, W. T. (2008). Tobacco use and cessation in psychiatric disorders: National Institute of Mental Health report. *Nicotine Tobacco Research, 10*(12), 1691–1715. https://doi.org/10.1080/14622200802443569

Index

For the benefit of digital users, indexed terms that span two pages (e.g., 52–53) may, on occasion, appear on only one of those pages.

Figures are indicated by f following the page number